REALLY
GOOD
F WORDS

REALLY
GOOD
F WORDS

Your Interactive Guide to Self-Care

LORRIE FORDE

Book Cover Design: Marla Thompson
Editor: Nina Shoroplova
Assistant Editor: Susan Kehoe
Production Editor: Jennifer Kaleta
Typeset: Greg Salisbury
Portrait Photographer: Spencer Kovats

DISCLAIMER: This book is a guide intended to offer information on how to connect with oneself and others. It is not intended in any way to replace other professional health care or mental health advice, but to support it. Readers of this publication agree that neither the author nor her publisher will be held responsible or liable for damages that may be alleged or resulting directly or indirectly from the reading of this publication.

This dedication is focused on two Really Good F Words.

The first is Family. To my mom and dad, Bob and Lorna Forde, who modeled healthy self-care at the same time as they provided an ideal home for my sister Karen, two brothers Rob and John, and me. To my children, Dean and Lani, who not only survived but thrived as they spent their lives watching me stretch and grow with my own self-care practice and who today are two of the most amazing people I know. And to my grandchildren, Corbin, Kingston, and Danyka, all my nieces and nephews, and the Family that is yet to be born—may you carry this torch of intentional self-care proudly into the future with you.

The second F word is Freedom. That we live in a place where we are free to talk about intentionally growing our personal self-care practice leaves me unbelievably grateful. My daughter-in-law, Monique gave me a magnet in the shape of the word Freedom for Mother's Day this year. It now holds a special place on the front of my fridge where I post my favourite photo or a meaningful quote. That magnet is not only functional in its purpose but it also provides me with a great reminder of this gift I am so thankful for each and every day.

Testimonials

"Lorrie Forde's book Really Good F Words is a brilliant approach to helping people who want more than just lip service when they are motivated to move forward in their lives. This book is not only well written, it gives you simple, real life examples and then has you thinking and writing as you move into your own 'stuff', coming out the other end more aware and energized. Congratulations Lorrie on a transformational book."
Linda Edgecombe: CSP - Hall of Fame Speaker - Author

"Really Good F Words is filled with inspirational moments and is an incredible read. Life-changing, readable, thought provoking, and an easy path to navigate in pursuit of self-care or any goal a reader sets their sights on."
Mohini Singh: Order of British Columbia (2008)
Kelowna City Councillor - former TV and CBC Radio journalist.

"I believe that you will discover in Lorrie Forde's words a combination of practical insight and experiences that characterizes my experience of her as an Executive and Life Coach. Perhaps most importantly she brings to life in these pages her unique combination of edge and compassion for others as we seek that seemingly elusive balance in our lives. I've personally experienced many of Lorrie's F words and trust that you will be motivated and inspired like I was to stay in balance and live with purpose."
Greg Hadubiak: Executive Coach
TEC Canada Chair – Consultant - Speaker

"Lorrie Forde is an enthusiastic and affectionate coach. Reading this book is like sitting around the kitchen table talking with a patient friend."
Francie Greenslade: Author – English Professor

Acknowledgements

Just as it takes a village to raise a child, so does it take a lot of people to get a book about really good F words to print!

Special thanks to Lynda Green, my sister/friend of more than thirty-five years, who is really the boot behind the kick that got me started along this Really Good F Word journey. Your initial encouragement and ongoing support have not gone un-noticed amiga.

There have been many contributors and supporters along the way. In addition to all those men and women who opened up to me during my research phase and provided me with candid responses, stories, and information I'd like to extend special appreciation to Laurie McDaniel, Jade Loan, Kimberley Mackereth, Anita Bakker, Tanya Swaren, Joseph Seiler, Maja Karlsson, Judi Wallace, Adonica Sweet, and Shawna McCrea who are just a few of the VIP's who helped me to bring this book to life. Thanks to you all!

And the team at Influence Publishing is deserving of mention here too. Thanks to my amazing editor Nina Shoroplova, Influence founder and owner Julie Salisbury who guides the ship, and the team in the office of Lyda Mclallen and Lisa Halpern who look after all things marketing and administration as they juggle their many authors.

You too dear reader, I'd like to acknowledge you and the fact that you have chosen to embark on this path to enhanced and intentional self-care through Really Good F Words. Thank you for giving my book your valuable time and consideration.

"Self-care is the heartbeat of living a balanced life and the answer to accomplishing everything that you want to do."
Lorrie Forde

Contents

Preface

When I was eighteen and just out of high school I had the world by the tail and never in a million years thought that I'd hear myself say, "If only I had known then what I know now." As I write this from my vantage point of nearing the sixty-year mark, I can assure you that I have heard myself say those very words. My intention is that by offering you this peek behind the curtain of life's learning (mine and others') at the same time as you're engaged in the coaching activities spread throughout this book, you'll be well-positioned to be pre-emptive and avoid those words too.

My **Family** of origin was by all accounts perfect. I am the eldest of four (two girls and two boys), my parents were loving and supportive, disputes were met with healthy communication, and respect was the **Foundation** of daily life. This was a wonderful reality to grow up in and I was well equipped to go **Forward** with my life. At the same time, I was a little naive and therefore ill-prepared for the realities of a world where some people cannot be trusted, healthy communication is not always the norm, and respectful behaviours are not guaranteed.

Marriage to my Prince Charming at twenty and having two kids (a son and a daughter) by age twenty-four were the beginning of a storybook life. Unfortunately, my story didn't have the happy ending I'd envisioned as it began. Divorced and a single parent of two pre-teens by thirty-five meant that there were emotional challenges and financial struggles I had not foreseen. Still today, all these years later, I can recall the sadness and loneliness I **Felt** during those early days of separation and divorce. Those memories are no longer sad though—today I recognize them as powerful lessons and, in truth, while I may not literally smile at the recall, I have a feeling of gratitude and a light-hearted appreciation for the fact that my Prince Charming gave me all he had to give. He gave me two wonderful children and he provided me with the opportunity to gain a perspective that brought some balance to the "Pollyanna" viewpoint I'd had until then.

There were several months when I was pretty low though, and there were two events during that time that I credit as being pivotal in shifting me from the low I was currently experiencing to a much healthier perspective—a vantage point where I could begin to see things as they really were.

The **First** was a VHS video (yes, it was that long ago—that was the technology of the day) given to me by one of my brothers. The video's message was that there is incredible power in the art of re-languaging or reframing the words we use in support of an intentional goal. I'd been **Feeling** very sorry for myself when I decided that something needed to change. My plan of action would be that any time I was going to undertake anything I would re-language my words to be, "I'm doing this or that *with* myself" as opposed to "*by* myself." The move from "by" to "with" was powerful for me and I've never looked back. I could **Feel** myself shifting from victim to the person in charge and it **Felt** great!

The second critical event was when my parents surprised me with a very special party for my thirty-sixth birthday. They hosted this party at the Fraser Downs Racetrack and Casino in Cloverdale, British Columbia. It was a night filled with **Fun**! The excitement of the horse races, the thrill when a bet paid off, and the **Feeling** that comes with knowing you're among people who love you so much that they're happy to create such a special memory for you. The proverbial icing on my birthday cake that evening was when the tenth race (my birthday is on the tenth day of the tenth month) was announced as the Lorrie Mae Classic. I was officially the dignitary for the race and as such was welcomed into the Winners Circle (along with my kids) to join the owners, the winning horse, and his jockey for photos. I couldn't remember the last time I'd **Felt** so honoured and again—I literally sensed the shift. I was moving from sad to happy, from empty to **Full**, and from **Feeling** weak to **Feeling** strong.

All in all, I've come through times when my self-care practices were poor at best and I've also ridden the high of being intentional about looking after myself on a daily basis. My hope for you is that you'll find your load lightened and your life journey made easier by the **Fact** that you've read this book, found empathy on its pages, and become intentional about your own self-care practice through the activities and assignments you're invited to complete.

Pivotal moments such as the two I described—the support of **Family** and **Friends**, and my own desire and willingness to move to a better place—created the path I took to getting where I am today. You'll learn more about that as we move **Forward**, so for now, I'll just say, "Welcome, and I look **Forward** to spending time with you."

The journey of travelling through the pages of this book will take you past a few really great **F** words, give you an opportunity to consider the **Fact** that self-care is NOT selfish, and provide you with a sneak peek into some stories from my colleagues, my clients, and my own personal experiences. In my Mountaintop Coaching practice as a Certified Executive Coach (mountaintop-coaching.ca), I've come to know that self-care is a skill and, as is the case with all skills, it requires ongoing commitment and practice.

You may already be wondering what makes one **F** word really good and another one not as good. For me, **F** words can be defined as good when the **Feeling** that **Follows** them is also good. Words like **Family** and **Friends** are pretty obvious yet when it comes to words like "**First**" and "**Follow**," it may not be quite as easy to see why they're highlighted. I choose to make **First** a really good **F** word because it leaves me with the **Feeling** of having just taken a step in a particular direction. The direction may or may not be great; however, the **Fact** that I've taken a step in any direction **Feels** good. If "**Follow**" is also ambiguous for you, think of a time when you've talked about **Following** through on something or when you think about **Following** your dreams. **Feels** pretty good when you put it that way, doesn't it? How about **Fact**? Do you think **Fact** deserves to be a really good **F** word? When I consider the **Facts**, it reminds me about the truth and I always **Feel** good knowing the truth about something. Whichever **F** word you're looking at, remember that you get to choose whether it's a good one or not. Remember too that there may be times that an **F** words shifts from good to bad or bad to good. It's all about how it leaves you **Feeling**.

Please consider this book an invitation to engage in an exciting journey toward self-care as this may be one of the most important topics we face in the twenty-first century. Stressors are at an all-time high and people are falling through the cracks of life. Perhaps *Really Good F Words* and the self-care it calls us to practise will be significant enough to be considered a crusade or a movement when our children and grandchildren look back in time. Regardless of the designation it is given, it will impact the reality of all who subscribe. This movement is **Focused** on strategizing for self-care in an intentional way. By accepting this invitation, you're saying "yes" to yourself. For some of you, that stance might **Feel** a little selfish. Don't worry, it's not; and we'll spend some time considering the question of where self-care crosses over into selfishness on the pages to come.

If the book looks like a lot of work—it is—and you're worth it. More than work, it's meant to be **Fun** and in support of you and your self-care practice. Plan to take your time working through the pages—there is no rush. If you're worried that you don't have time right now—that's okay too. You can choose to just flip through the pages and skim the chapters that jump out at you until you're ready to sink your teeth into the meat of it. It's your book and you're the boss so you get to decide how best you'd like to proceed. Having said that, I will add that there is a natural **Flow** to the book and it has been designed with your success in mind, so when you're ready to truly commit to growing or deepening your self-care practice, start at the beginning and let me be your guide. As we move into and through the pages of this interactive book, I will encourage and invite you to build your own community of support, to engage your **Friends** and **Family**, and to have **Fun** while you do it. In **Fact** , by the time you get midway through this book you'll be thriving in your customized community of **Friends** who are just as dedicated to growing through self-care as you are.

Based on the **Fact** that this book has found its way into your hands, I'm going to move **Forward** with the assumption that you're interested in and open to growing the notion of self-care in your own life. To that end, I have created an example of a to-do list (below) that might look like one you've written for yourself at some point. Please **Feel Free** to adjust it however you like so the words sound like your own. Consider it a starting point. It might be your resolution for the year ahead or it could be a promise or a wish for change that you're making at a time when you're facing one of those pivotal moments where you just *know* that something needs to change.

> *My Goal: Healthy Self-Care with lots of Fun and Friends*
> *Barriers to Achieving My Goal: Life, Work, Everything …*
> *My Self-Care Plan: I don't even know where to start and I Feel like it's just one more thing on my never-ending list of things to do.*

Does this to-do list look familiar? You're not alone.

We've all written goals for ourselves—this time will be a little different. You're going to have the support of the structure of this interactive book to help you turn your goal of healthy self-care into reality. The categories in this to-do list are simply the shorthand version of where this book will take you. In the beginning, you'll have a goal; there will be barriers along the way and, by the end, you will have a doable plan of action to achieve your goal.

Allow me to join you on this journey as your personal coach. You'll see notes like this from me throughout the pages of this book. You'll recognize them as they'll be written in this same font. It will be as though I'm right here in the room with you. As we move through the pages, we'll work toward believing that self-care is not selfish as we use some really good 'F' words to have some *Fun* at the same time. For me, *Fun* and laughter are a big part of self-care. I know I always *Feel* lighter and brighter when I've had a good belly laugh or enjoyed some *Fun* activity with a *Friend*. We must share that quality—you and I—you picked up a book with a title that certainly made me laugh the *First* time I saw it in print. The title also invites curiosity and I encourage you to draw on the curious part of yourself as you move through these pages with me.

Lorrie

CHAPTER
1

THE GROUNDWORK

- Did the title of this book catch your attention?
- Are you **Feeling** the need for some self-care?
- Are you wondering if the **F** words you've been using fall under the heading of *good*?
- Have you read a million self-help books and you're wondering if this one will be different?
- Are you looking for ideas on how to turn mayhem into me-time?
- Did you hear about the book from a **Friend**?
- Do you know someone you'd like to gift this book to?

Whatever the reason—Congratulations and welcome. This book is different: it will call you to action. You're not just picking up a book; you're taking on a personal coach and moving in the direction of gaining a community of support where like-minded people are willing to have **Fun** while they maintain **Forward-Focused** momentum. Throughout the pages of this book, you will be asked to answer a variety of questions. There is method to the madness—it's all in aid of and designed for developing a plan to support a healthy practice of self-care. Nine of the questions will be framed as personal assignments and fourteen will be called group activities. Plan to work through these personal assignments on your own in a place where you have the space and time to **Focus**. The group activities are all about interacting and having **Fun** with a group of **Friends**, your customized community of support. While you're working through these activities, you'll also be learning more about yourself through the coach-like conversations that will be a part of each activity. All of the assignments and activities are in support of your moving in the direction of your own self-care practice. Set yourself up for success. Don't rush, enjoy the process, and stay present in the journey of exploring the adventure that is *Really Good F Words*. Allow me (and this book) to be your coach along the way.

Coaches help create a perfect storm for their clients. A coach's perfect storm is where interest and desire meet planning, preparation, and commitment to action. My questions will open the door to your answers, and those answers will inform your next steps as you strategize for success in achieving your self-care goal(s).

As I've already mentioned earlier, people often **Feel** worried that their self-care will appear selfish. It's an interesting point to ponder. I believe most of us intuitively know the difference between "self-care" and "selfishness" when we're in the moment with either, but that difference can be challenging to explain. I'm confident that I know when I cross the line. When asked by a young man the other day if I could give a definition in support of a deeper understanding between the two, I had to stop and think. In the end, I decided my best explanation was to parallel "self-care" with assertiveness and "selfishness" with aggression. Just as behaving in an assertive way takes care of your own interests without stepping on the interests of another, so self-care takes care of your needs without stepping on the needs of another. Aggressive behaviour also takes care of your interests; however, it does so at the expense of another person's. In the same way, selfish behaviour takes care of your needs at the expense of another's. As you consider your own awareness on that topic and difference between the terms, here's a little visual that speaks to the theme.

Imagine yourself at a dinner event (perhaps it's a wedding). It's a self-serve buffet and you're starving! Your stomach is making awful noises and your hypoglycemic symptoms are beginning to appear. You can **Feel** yourself becoming agitated and all you want is something to eat—it's one of those scenes from a movie where the "crazy you" is minutes away from appearing.

Do you:

A) walk quietly and discreetly to the **Food** table where you can get a piece of cheese and a cracker before going back to the end of the line?
OR
B) push your way **Forward**, demanding you move to the front of the line NOW?

I've chosen this very visual image as it conjures up a **Funny** picture, and according to its title, this book is about really good **F** words after all. As well, I think the image makes it easy to see which option leans further in the direction of self-care and which tends more toward the classic selfish or self-centered behaviour that we all recognize as offensive and something to avoid.

The bottom line on this question is that, like most things, it's a personal choice. Only you can determine where self-care ends and selfishness begins. I like to think of it as a spectrum or a continuum with martyrdom at one end and over the top self-serving selfishness at the other. I strive for balance every day as I move along this line with each choice I make. My target is always somewhere near the middle, where healthy self-care stands proud and tall. Like any skill, practise makes perfect, so practise, practise, practise, and before you know it, it will be second nature.

F words typically have a negative connotation attached to them. Let's challenge that belief! Before we go too far down that road, let us **First** take a minute to set the stage and conjure up a couple of images that draw out our empathic responses. The goal here is that everyone who has picked up this book will enter into it with a similar definition of what self-care is and why we might want it.

Many times, I've seen people shake their heads in judgement. In **Fact**, I can even think of a few times when I've been the person shaking my head. Can you recall any times when you've seen someone appear to judge another? How about a time when you've been the judger? Or the person being judged?

One example of a time that I went straight to judging took place just the other day when I noticed a young mom in the park on her cell phone while her kids were clearly calling out for her attention. I remember my **First** thought was that she is obviously more interested in her cell phone than in taking care of her kids. Right behind that thought were some of my judgements about the overuse of technology, parenting (or lack of parenting to be more exact), screaming kids, and … I'm sure you get the picture.

How about this second image in a shoe store? There are a few shoppers taking advantage of an end-of-season sale in the store. Off to one side are a young woman and a girl, likely mother and daughter, sitting on a bench. Another person in the store is a woman who is waiting for the sales clerk to finish with her current customer so she can get some service too. This woman is watching the mother and daughter duo on the bench and as she does she heaves a sigh of disdain as the young mom says "no" to her daughter's plea for a new pair of runners while choosing a pair of strappy sandals for herself instead. Can you imagine how it might **Feel** to be either the woman buying the sandals or the person heaving the sigh?

None of us can know someone else's story. We may know bits and pieces of it, but we cannot know everything about it. The day of the week, the weather, the thing that happened just seconds before all factors into the way we respond to what's happening around us. It was unfair of me to judge the young mom on her cell phone in the park. I will never know whom she was speaking with. Perhaps it was her doctor's office and she was getting the results from her follow-up mammogram. Maybe it was her sister who was in tears and needing attention more than the kids did. I could come up with a million different scenarios and none of them would be exactly right.

What about the woman who sighed as she judged the other woman in the shoe store? I'm almost certain she will never find out that those strappy sandals are a birthday gift and for a special event the young woman purchasing them is nervous about attending. Chances are good that the woman will never know the young mom also doesn't want to spoil her daughter's surprise when her dad takes her on a special date that upcoming weekend, a date where part of the plan is to go shopping for runners.

Now try to think of a time that you've **Felt** judged for taking a minute to do something for yourself. The purpose of this exercise is not to go back there and dwell on the negative **Feelings** that being judged can promote. More importantly, it is to recognize that judgement can get in the way of self-care. It is through this type of awareness that we will find the motivation to begin the journey **Forward** toward a commitment to practising regular self-care. We will also gain a new clarity about what self-care looks like for each of us. Just as we all have unique interests and preferences, the self-care strategies that speak to us are also unique. Mine will be different from yours and yours will be different from your neighbour's.

Whatever our story, each of us is unique and deserving of self-care. By turning the world on its head, inviting the use of some really good **F** words, and committing to making those **F** words work for us in our day-to-day lives—we will be well on our way to making self-care part of our daily regime.

Here is a story one of my clients recently shared with me and gave me permission to include in this book. It is a story I suspect many of you will be able to relate to on some level. It's a tale that speaks to the value of practising healthy self-care at the same time as it is a great example of how the best-laid plans can go awry. This is a story in which I think it would have been really easy to utter some of those not-so-good *F* words!

Maggie's Story

It was ten to seven on Friday night. I'd been waiting all week for this moment. My husband and I had a deal where this night would be his turn to put the kids to bed, looking after all the washing of bodies, brushing of teeth and hair, reading of stories, and inevitable miscellaneous delays that that task generally entails.

This week had been a long one for me. Work had been more demanding than usual and I was pretty sure my five-year-old was hitting puberty! The drama and emotions that seemed to have overtaken my sweet little girl were wearing thin on me and I knew instinctively that I was due for some me-time.

I'm pretty good at taking time for myself, yet that wasn't always the case. There was a time when I didn't even know what self-care was, let alone how to practise it. In **Fact**, I'm positive it is thanks to my commitment to taking regular time for myself that I'm smiling at the memory of this story. Had I not been so intentional with that practice of regular self-care for a long time now, this story might have had a very different ending.

My husband was outside tinkering with his car. Men are good like that. They know how to take time to do the things they enjoy. I often watch to see how he does it—how he creates space for himself—what he says—how he moves to action. In truth, once, I even took notes! I digress; that's another story entirely.

So here we are at the end of a very long week. I've been waiting for Friday at seven because that's the time I've set aside to run a hot bath—you know the kind—hard to get into and once you do you literally melt. Waiting all week to sink into the lavender-scented suds with a book I've been dying to read, and to stay there till the water turns cool, and my skin is so saturated it goes all wrinkly.

I called out to my husband to give him the ten-minute sign, and he smiled as he nodded and said, "I'll be right there."

At that moment, I knew my life was good. My husband is the best and I'm on my way to my **Favourite** place: a hot bath with a great book. Everything was right in my world!

Within ten minutes, my husband was well-entrenched in prepping the kids for bed. I could hear him responding to their protests and questions in his calm quiet way. My bath was running and the lavender-scented bubbles were billowing up and threatening to spill over the edge of the tub and onto the floor.

It seemed odd that the bathroom wasn't steamy. I had left the door open and the window wasn't closed either—maybe that was why. I lit a candle, grabbed my book, and prepared to dip my toes into the blessed warmth that promised to absorb my week's stress.

You can't imagine my distress and the cruel shock I **Felt** when my toes were met with frigid icy water. There couldn't be a drop of hot in the tub—in **Fact**, it **Felt** as though the water had been shipped in directly from some glacial stream!

I turned on the hot tap in the sink only to be met with more of the icy cold liquid. I think it was at that moment when the beginning of a sick **Feeling** began to dawn in the pit of my stomach. Something was very, very wrong!

I pulled my dirty clothes back on and crept down the stairs to the basement area we'd been promising ourselves we would do something with for years. By the time I was halfway down the stairs, I could see what had happened. The hot water tank had sprung a leak and spilled its entire contents throughout the basement. I speculated whether the easy answer might be to turn the basement into a pool. I wondered if the water on the floor was still warm enough to bathe in. I sat on the stairs and **Felt** like that old A.A. Milne story about a boy, Christopher Robin, who sits on a stair that is halfway up and halfway down. I thought about how strange it was that I was remembering an old story from my childhood and that's when I began to laugh. My blissful bath hadn't worked out as planned and here I was laughing like a crazy person. I could literally **Feel** my stress melting away. I realized I might not get much me-time this weekend and I also knew that I could choose to see this bath-gone-wrong as the opportunity it was. This would be the motivation we'd been waiting for to spur us to action on our basement.

As I said earlier, I'm positive that my regular practice of self-care set me up to be able to find the **Funny** side of this scenario. Being tired after a long week of work isn't nearly as bad as being a walking zombie after too many long weeks without time for self-care. Because I had been taking care of myself on a regular basis, I was able to laugh as I saw past the horror and all the way to the opportunity this flooded basement could provide.

Sitting there with nothing other than a torrent of tears and a sense of sinking deeper under the veil of exhaustion was how I might have responded to the situation a year or two earlier. Now, however, I had the strength and perspective to see the possibilities more clearly than the problems.

I could go on—but in the end—we have a new hot water tank, the kids are having Fun in their new playroom, and I'm heading into a luxuriously HOT bubble bath as I finish writing this recap.

For me, self-care is critical to my ability to take care of my **Family** and other responsibilities. As I recount this story, I can see that it also provides me with the perspective to be able to laugh in the face of adversity and I LOVE TO LAUGH!

Maggie was able to find the _Fun_ and the _Funny_. In her story, she does a great job of recognizing that her routine of blocking off time for herself put her in good stead for being able to face adversity when it hit.

As I read over Maggie's story, I am especially struck by her final comment about the Fact that she loves to laugh. While she references a memory from her youth about Christopher Robin, I'm propelled back to one of my own childhood memories to recall a specific song and a scene from Disney's 1964 movie _Mary Poppins._ The song is "I Love to Laugh" (composers Richard M. Sherman and Robert B. Sherman) and the scene depicts laughter as the infectious element that provides the person who is laughing with a joyous power that enables them to float high above the rest of the world. If you've never had the opportunity to experience the magic that is Mary Poppins, I encourage you to take the time to watch this timeless classic. My wager is that you'll find the laughter in this scene and this song so contagious that you will walk away humming that you "love to laugh," and the child in you will wonder if it might really be possible to _Fly_.

"The most wasted day is one without laughter."
E.E. Cummings

WELCOME TO MY SELF-CARE CLUB

We're all in this together and this book will be a tool we use to keep us **Focused** and moving **Forward** in the direction of a commitment to regular self-care. We live in a world where demands are great and time can seem like an elusive luxury. The chapters and the activities in this interactive, light-hearted, and insightful book will invite and encourage you to lighten up the topic of strategizing for self-care by using some of those really good F words. Making something **Fun** helps me stay motivated and on track, and I know that when I see my **Friends** having **Fun**, I want to join them. Committing to take the time to **Focus** on anything is a powerful step in getting clear on where I'd like to go and that clarity helps me plan my strategy for action, a sure way for anyone wanting to reach a specific destination.

In keeping with the words "**Fun, Friends, Forward**," and "**Focused**," and given that I just welcomed you to my "club," I am going to introduce one **Fun** element here that I believe will provide us with some language to use later in the book as we dig deeper into the concept of strategizing for self-care. This quick peek at the **Fun** element I refer to is all about cookies—and who doesn't love cookies? Don't worry, there are no calories in these cookies. They're imaginary—just an analogy. I'll be asking you to consider using cookies and a cookie jar as concepts that are intended to support you as you move toward an intentional self-care regime. A couple of chapters further along the journey of these pages you will create customized strategies for **Filling** your "cookie jar," an action plan to keep you on track, and an accountability process that will support you through those times when it **Feels** like there is no time or energy for anything—not even cookies!

In my work as a coach and in my day-to-day life as a grandma, a mom, a sister, a daughter, and a **Friend**, I have seen time and again that we're not very good at taking care of ourselves. Women in particular are hard-wired to put others **First**. While men too will benefit from exploring their own cookie jars, this book is written with women in mind—particularly young moms who are working at juggling it all. Whether you decide to work with **Friends** or on your own, exploring this cookie jar concept will be **Fun, Fact-Filled, Focused**, and **Freeing**. You will be in the driver's seat as we explore how often you bake, how **Full** (or empty) your jar is when you bake, what kind of a baker you are, whether you leave the lid off your jar inviting any and all to help themselves as they choose, or if you're cautious about sharing your cookies and why that might be.

Courage, intention, authenticity, curiosity, compassion, and an open mind will all serve you well as you embark on this journey into a land where your self-care is the theme and you are both the author and the star of the show. **Fun** and **Friends** are two of the really good **F** words that will make your journey memorable.

If we were meeting face to face, I'd promise to be your confidential non-judgemental thinking partner and, even though we're meeting in print, I can still commit to being that. As your coach, I believe that you have all your own best answers and that it is my job to coax those answers out of you with some really good questions. These questions are always moving in the direction of your goal(s). I'll ask you to write things down, to talk about your "ahas" with trusted **Friends** and allies, and to reflect back over the experience that this interactive book invites. As you read back over your own notes and hear the stories of others, use your natural creative curiosity to think of what

I might ask you about your self-judgement, your perspective, your level of open-mindedness, and your willingness to move **Forward** toward your goal(s). Remember those key elements of being confidential and non-judgemental—be as kind to yourself and any others you choose to share this experience with as I'd be with you.

In parts of this book there will be a lot more of me than there is of you, and by the end, you will see that there are also sections where there is a lot more of you than there is of me. Coaching is based in the belief that we all have our own best answers. When it's your words and your ideas you'll **Feel** more motivated to **Follow** through to action and having you reach your goal is my goal in writing this book.

Glossary of Terms

- Coach—A non-judgemental confidential thinking partner.
- **F Words**—We will **Focus** on the "good ones" throughout this book.
- Cookie Jar—You.
- Baking Cookies—Self-Care Strategies.
- Cookies—Health, happiness, balance, or whatever you'd like them to be.
- Barriers—Nothing more than hurdles along the path leading to achieving your goal.

Before we delve further into the analogy of the cookie jar and strategizing for your self-care, I invite you to spend the next few pages getting to know me a little better and allowing me to divulge some of the learning that has come my way. In these pages, I'll also invite you to ask yourself some interesting questions. All of them are in support of growing your self-care practices, so dive in and give it a hundred percent because you're worth it! Much of what you'll read in this book came to me by way of my life's journey and my formal education, some of it via the interviews I did as part of the research for this book, and the rest of it as a gift from a few courageous folk who were willing to share their own personal stories. (The earlier story from Maggie was from one of those people brave enough to give me permission to share their account in this book.) The stories are real and the names are fictitious.

CHAPTER

3

CURVEBALLS CAN CHANGE A GAME

My work in post-secondary education was well into its twenty-fourth year when a curveball changed my game. I had a great career, I loved my work, and I knew how **Fortunate** I was to have such a good job. I was engaged and involved at a variety of levels within the organization and I knew I was doing some really important work. I was making a difference in the lives of many and knowing that provided me with a sense of purpose that made the long hours and occasional challenges worthwhile.

At the same time, I was aware that many of my tasks had become mundane and that a sense of lethargy hung like a cloud over my desk. So much of the **Fun** was gone. Each day I pushed that cloud aside and **Focused** on the elements of my work that I loved.

One of those **Favourite** duties was working directly with students enrolled in the institution. I was **Fully** engaged in working closely with a group of students who were attending a program that supported them to **Focus** on overcoming personal and employment barriers; they were earning a credential that would enable them to work in a field connected with their career interests. Every day was exciting for me as I watched the students advance toward their personal journeys of learning, education, and growth. It was also rewarding as I knew that my role in their experience was valued and valuable. I **Felt** a kindred spirit with each of them and as with many experiences one or two students stood out.

I **Felt** proud for each of them on their final day as they stood to receive their credentials and congratulations from the crowd that had gathered for the graduation event. It was exciting to hear the graduates describe their next steps and rewarding to see their passion, enthusiasm, and new confidence. One student in particular made my heart sing—he was twenty-seven years old, he had overcome significant barriers, and he had committed to returning to college to pursue the higher learning that would connect him to his "heart's desire."

Just ten days later that curveball I refer to in the title of this chapter hit me **Full** force. For no apparent reason this same young man's heart stopped beating—it just stopped—and he was gone. When the report came in about his sudden death, I didn't recognize the curveball for what it was. That recognition came a few days later, during his funeral. Sometime after the **Fact**, I would describe it to **Friends** as "**Feeling** as though I'd been hit on the side of my head with a two-by-four." I knew in that moment, during his funeral, that life deserves to be **Fully** lived with passion at its centre. This young man who had so recently unlocked his own driving force as he **Focused** on opening doors to his purpose had been ripped away. Too much of what I was spending so many hours a day on was no longer connected with who I am at my core and that **Fact** was suddenly crystal clear and screaming at me. It was a lesson that I'd learned before and from which I had somehow drifted away. The time had come for me to dial back in for clarity and—in keeping with the analogy of the curveball—to swing for the fence—to go for the home run that could change the game.

It was important to me that I treat this change with the attention it deserved. I committed to giving myself as much time as I needed. I would explore all the pros and cons, and seek out support that would help me make a decision that would be the best for me, my **Future**, and my need for connection with purposeful work. I worked with my coach and also took the time to see a counsellor. I accessed the wisdom of others who had walked the path of change before me, **Friends** became my sounding board, and I "baked a lot of cookies."

Four months later, I had my answer. I knew with all certainty that the time had come to say goodbye to the work I had done for almost twenty-five years. Goodbye at that time made no logical sense as I was less than two years away from a **Full** pension. I said goodbye to the job that had allowed me to provide for my **Family** as they grew from children to adults. I said goodbye to the position that provided excellent benefits, annual vacations, and great people to work with. I said goodbye to the job that had spilled over the edges and into my life to become a big part of who I was. Regardless of all that, my decision was crystal clear—I would retain and grow the parts of my work that I loved and leave the rest behind.

I returned to university for some graduate work where I elevated my coaching skills and credential to Certified Executive Coach, a designation that is internationally recognized, and that enables me to work in fields ranging from executive and business coaching to career and life coaching. By leaving behind the work that didn't resonate with my passion, I created the time and space to build a portfolio that included work which **Filled** me up—and that brings us to the place where that curveball connected with the birth of this book: it was a game-changing shift.

That's one part of my story—by the end of this book, you will have connected with at least one part of yours.

> *You may have noticed in this story, that for a while I'd lost sight of a few of those really good F words. Fortunately for me, my life is Full of good F words again.*

"Getting knocked down in life is a given. Getting up and moving ***Forward*** *is a choice."*
Zig Ziglar

CHAPTER
4

BEATING THE BAD

De-mystifying the practice of self-care is a critical step in connecting with your passion and for moving to action in the quest to live a **Full** life. When I look at a maze from the starting point, I struggle with finding the best way through to the other end. When I adjust my perspective so I'm looking at the puzzle from that end point, the path is much clearer. That same tactic can work with finding the most direct path through the puzzle of life. By starting with the desired result in mind and knowing where I want to end up, I can look backward to easily identify potential hurdles and barriers along the way. By knowing where the hurdles and barriers are, I'm better able to plan for them, avoid them, and plot the shortest and most efficient route through the maze.

Consider your own healthy self-care practice as the end point of this maze. Think about the hurdles, negative influences, and potential supports you can see as you look back from that finish line. Practising self-care and **Filling** up on life is great in theory, and we've all experienced the negativity that can get in the way of our success. Sometimes the negativity is external but more often it is internal.

While external pessimism is difficult to manage, the internal disapproval is even more challenging. This is one of those times where the adage, "We're our own worst enemy," couldn't be truer. The internal negativity could be described as the little demon that sits on our shoulder challenging us, leaving us **Feeling** like "we don't deserve it" or that "we can't do it." In the maze, that little demon is represented by those hurdles, the barriers, and the negative voices and influences we'll face along the path of this puzzle. Using the maze analogy helps me get clear on the steps to take as I move in the direction of my self-care goal. As you read on, I invite you to consider how you can befriend that "little demon" and get it to work for you versus against you. Reframing negative thoughts into positive ones may seem like a daunting task; however, I assure you it is possible. Being intentional with any goal is the best way to accomplish it and through reframing your inner self-talk toward something more positive, supportive, and curious, you'll find yourself **Feeling** empowered and strong, willing to take on new projects, and as a result getting more of what you do want and less of what you don't.

This book is yours to do with as you like and I'm hoping that you'll play along with me and be okay with the **Fact** that I will be asking you to break all the old rules about not writing in books and to use it as your personal customized workbook. Take a minute right now and if you haven't already, grab a highlighter to capture text that has special meaning for you and pick up a pen so you can scribble in the margins and draw in the spaces. Plan to flip back and forth so you can revisit topics or activities as you think of more to add—**Feel Free** to use this workbook in **Fun** and interesting ways that will serve you in moving in the direction of strategizing for your self-care. Perhaps you will think of this book as a journal—something you can reflect on or refer back to in the **Future**. It's really just a vehicle to support you having an intentional conversation with yourself as you move in the direction of building your own unique community that **Focuses** on having **Fun** while supporting healthy self-care practices.

This is where you'll need that pen. Begin to get used to writing in your book—there will be more of these questions so dive in, have Fun , and enjoy this exercise in self-awareness. Self-awareness is step one in self-care.

How do you manage your negative self-talk when it rears its ugly head in your moments of self-doubt?

_____

_____

_____

_____

_____

Over the next few pages, we'll visit people who are willing to share their own experiences with their negative self-talk (the "little demon" that sits on their shoulder) and what they do to manage it. Perhaps you'll recognize some strategies in their stories that you can use to help you as you work toward solving your own puzzle. You'll see that some people refer to their negative self-talk as "it," while others call it a "gremlin." The common denominator is that we all face this "little demon" at different times in our lives so know that you're not alone and that you're already well on your way to managing your negative self-talk.

> *"Don't say anything about yourself that you*
> *wouldn't say about your best Friend."*
> **Lorrie Forde**

My Story

As is the case for many of us, my own personal style has evolved over the years. Today I can confidently say that my chosen response to negative self-talk is to comfortably reframe negatives into positives and challenges into opportunities. Much of the reason for my ability to manage negative self-talk today is due to my ongoing commitment to living a balanced life in which stressors are minimized and self-care is a daily practice. However, it was not always that way for me and occasionally I find myself back in a place where I need to revisit what has worked for me in the past.

As I reflect on my life experience with negative self-talk, I can see that my style has always tended more to an intuitive fight-or-flight scenario and that generally I have been more susceptible to negative self-talk during times when I've been **Feeling** tired or overwhelmed. Most often I would choose to take on a fighting stance—I would look at my negative self-talk as a challenge to be beaten. That self-awareness, clarity of **Focus**, and the accompanying passion would provide me with the motivation to stay on track until I had moved past the negative self-talk into a place where I overcame hurdles and achieved my goals.

There were also those other times when I chose to flee and hide from that negative inner voice. It was during those times of hiding that I chose to call upon my logical self to remind me that I'm worth it, that I deserve to be able to decide which direction I want to go, and that I can do it this time just like I've done it before. Those were the times when I would draw on strategies such as:

- talking to someone I trust to gain new perspective or to build my confidence. This person might be my coach, a **Family** member, or someone from my circle of close **Friends** .
- popping a peppermint or a piece of gum into my mouth. As simple as that sounds, sometimes just the soothing aroma of peppermint and the act of taking the time to open the candy can calm my nerves and help me see my options a little more clearly.
- stepping away from the issue long enough to give myself some space and time to just breathe, which often helps me to calm down. (Even just a few minutes locked in the bathroom can do wonders!)
- giving myself a mini massage. There is a little spot just behind your ears and at the base of your skull that loves to be rubbed!
- intentionally thinking of times when I've beaten negative self-talk in the past and looking at how I was able to do it.
- embracing the "fake it till you make it" philosophy, as I've learned that the confidence to do something often doesn't come till after the doing is done and you can look back on the journey and see that you've lived to tell the tale.
- **Forgiving** myself if this is one of the times when, in the end, I choose not to move to action right now.

You may have noticed that I used the word *choose* when talking about my response to working with or managing my own negative self-talk. It's an important distinction. Everything we do is a choice. Choice equates to accepting responsibility for the outcome and at the same time, it brings the reward that is earned when we know we've taken ownership of something. It's not about taking on some kind of blame—it's about accepting responsibility for ourselves and the choices we are **Free** to make. Perhaps another way of saying this is that with the **Freedom** to choose comes the responsibility of choice. Sometimes the places I least want to go, or **Feel** the most uncomfortable in, turn out to be the richest places I've ever been when I give them a little time and attention.

Here are a few more personal stories from my colleagues and clients about how they manage the negative character that makes its way to their shoulder during times of self-doubt and low confidence. With the exception of this first story from Mary, all the rest are written in their own words and I believe that brings a powerful validity to them. Their courageous honesty as they share these personal examples speaks to their success at managing their negative self-talk. The writers of these stories come from all walks of life and represent a variety of demographic categories. Negative self-talk happens for everyone—it's all about how you respond to it, rather than wondering whether it exists.

Mary's Story

This long-time **Friend** of mine gave me permission to share a strategy that's been highly effective for her. In **Fact**, it's been so many years since her negative self-talk has gotten in the way of her moving **Forward** in a direction that she wanted to go that she wasn't even able to come up with a specific example of a recent time when she'd been seriously challenged. She literally talks to her "little fellow"—she gives him a name—and tells him to be patient for just a minute till she is finished doing whatever it is that he is trying to interrupt. Once she is finished with her planned action she goes back to the "little guy" only to discover he no longer has a voice as she has already done what he said she couldn't!

While this may sound overly simplistic, I can only tell you that I've seen first-hand that it works for her and—really—that is the only thing that matters: it works for her. Mary was happy to share her strategy in the hope that it may be as effective for others as she has found it to be.

This same **Friend** recalls a time in her life when she was not very good at practising healthy self-care. It was a time when her negative self-talk often got in the way of her ability to **Follow** through on things she wanted to do.

As with all things—practice makes perfect and she has been practising her strategy of managing negative self-talk for so long that she is now someone I would call a master of moving to action on her goals.

When I interviewed Terri during the research phase of this book, she was initially a little hesitant to put pen to paper and share her strategies. In the end though, she could hardly wait to tell me what a valuable exercise that had been for her. By taking the time to get really clear on how she manages her negative self-talk, she <u>Felt</u> she'd become even more effective in making her strategies work.

Terri's Story

Managing my own negative self-talk is something I take very seriously and I've discovered that when I incorporate a regular regime of self-care into my daily plan I'm better prepared to have success in all areas of my life. I know that stress may come at me from several different directions—work, **Family**, media, or the self-imposed "keeping up with the Joneses," so I'm committed to **Following** a plan of action that leaves me better prepared and **Feeling** powerful as I come face to face with those moments of self-doubt and negativity.

Each day,

- I take time to be quiet and reflective.
- I work toward staying intentionally present and **Focused** on "the now" versus worrying about what might happen.
- I **Forgive** myself.
- I am careful about the amount of negativity I expose myself to in the media, through the people I meet, and in the situations I face.
- I seek out and identify things and people who inspire me and encourage me to **Focus** on the positive.
- I look for ways to fulfill my intention of "being the change I want to see in the world" as I **Focus** on **Feeling** happy and healthy.

Investing in myself each and every day is the **Foundation** that supports me in achieving my goals without losing sight of the **Fact** that I can't be truly good to others until I'm truly good to myself.

Alice is a colleague who, as you'll see from her story, has been diligent as well as intentional in her practice of managing her own negative self-talk.

Alice's Story

When I first saw a posting for the position of Performance Coach, I was intrigued. My years in social work had left me **Feeling** like I was missing something. My personal mission to find a job that would provide me with the opportunity and the platform to bring out the best in others hadn't yet been achieved. Over the years, I had heard about the power of coaching as a skill and a strategy that could be used when supporting others to achieve their own goals with excellence. I **Felt** my excitement grow as I thought about the possibility of moving into the realm of coaching for performance and I knew I was hooked—I had to **Find** the courage to take the next steps.

Four years later, and now in hindsight, I can say that my natural skills had always enabled me to be coach-like in the work I did. Four years ago though, my gremlin was working overtime. He was telling me, "You are crazy" and "You can't do it," "You aren't certified as a coach," and "You don't know what you are doing!"

I listened to that gremlin and although I knew in my head that he was wrong on so many levels, I **Felt** the weight of his negativity. His pessimism did help me on one level though: it triggered me to begin the training I needed to become certified in the field of coaching AND, in so doing, to begin to recognize that I was headed in the right direction. I knew that I was on the right path my very **First** day in residency when I **Felt** as though I had come home. I was surrounded by like-minded people and the learning I was engaged in was a perfect fit with my personal style and my core values. Every day I was there, I could see the spark that was my interest burning more brightly as I worked hard to become an effective and credentialed coach.

During that time, my gremlin reared his head a number of times. He started with, "You can't go back to school! It's too much money and you work full-time."

I countered by researching schools to find one that accommodates students who have demanding careers.

His next attack **Focused** on the finances. "You're just going to go further into debt—you'll never get the money you need."

My response was to apply for and win a scholarship that covered half the cost. A student loan and frugal choices on all fronts took care of the other half.

"How are you going to go to school, work full time, and take care of your **Family?**"

This one was the most difficult—my cookie jar was empty much of the time. I used my dampened finger to pick up whatever crumbs I could find at the bottom of the jar, and when I was ready to give up because it was all just too much—here's what got me through:

- remaining as positive as I could—looking at my glass as half **Full** instead of half empty.
- connecting with others and sharing the burden. I worked with my own coach. I talked to my husband, classmates, supervisor, and colleagues.
- celebrating myself at every opportunity.

I was hard on myself, and that gremlin was on my shoulder all the time. I had to learn to let go of my need for perfection, to do homework in a storage room where I could find the quiet I needed, to be okay with living in a messy house, and to accept the **Fact** that I couldn't be all things to all people all the time. I learned so much about myself during that time.

Eventually I graduated as an executive coach and even though I continued to work full-time, I mustered the confidence to start my own business.

Still the gremlin remained ever present on my shoulder. This time his comments included: "You're never going to coach full-time." "Businesses take forever to build; you'll never get enough clients." "That position for a performance coach that started you down this path will never be posted again." And "You'll be stuck in this same old job forever."

I decided to draw on my previous experience and success in dealing with this negative gremlin.

I committed to believing in myself and my ability to achieve my goals. I said, "I will be a full-time coach!" The spark turned into an ember that I could **Feel** warm me at my core. My belief deepened as I continued with my mantra of becoming a full-time coach and I knew that I was **Following** my life's purpose—I was on the right path.

One year later, the position of performance coach was again posted. I applied for the job and am proud to say that I was the successful candidate. Today, I am living my life's purpose and I continue to overcome the negativity that gremlin decides to dump on me by **Following** the steps that served me well in getting to where I am today.

> *Sharry's example may seem almost too basic. Often it is those simple ideas that work the best and are the most sustainable.*

Sharry's Story

It seemed I was my own worst enemy on every front until one day I'd just simply had enough—I guess I hit that proverbial bottom people often refer to. I'm not sure what gave me the courage or the deep commitment it took for me to keep moving **Forward** over the months that followed. I did it though; and as a result, I'm able to tell this story today.

In the largest font I could fit onto a piece of paper, I printed an affirmation that I posted on my bedroom mirror; it said, "TODAY IS MY BEST DAY." Each morning that was the **First** thing I saw when I got up, and it was the last thing I saw before I went to bed at night. Every time I saw it, I said it aloud too.

In the beginning, it was really hard to say and I didn't believe it at all. I could hear my inner voices howling with laughter as I **Felt** my self-confidence shrivel. In spite of those inner voices, I continued to repeat the affirmation to the image I saw reflected in the mirror.

It took two long years and during that time the affirmation became easier to say aloud and the inner voices grew quieter. The piece of paper has since been removed from my mirror and yet I still say the same message to myself whenever I look at my reflection and today I believe it with all my heart. Today is my best day!

I knew the instant I read Jayne's story that I had to make room for it in this book. Jayne, like many of us, has met her challenges with courage and an open mind.

Jayne's Story

Rather than personalize it, my preference is to refer to the character that rears itself in moments of self-doubt as an "it," because "it," in my view, is just a pattern—a habitual way of thinking that runs mechanically in order to get "its" needs met. "It" never does though, because the needs are never-ending and cannot be fulfilled. I've spent a lifetime learning how to manage this negative force and will continue to do this important personal work because I know that I'm worth it.

Staying present and intentionally coming into awareness when "it" is up and running are the **Foundation** of my work. That **Focused** awareness helps me to *not* believe the story "it" is telling me about myself or others. I try not to be swallowed up by the story and **Feelings** that rise up and jeopardize my ability to stay present and aware during the triggers "it" pushes masterfully. The story line could be anything from "Nobody loves me—everyone hates me" to "I'm a terrible person," or

"Life is a struggle and I'll never get anywhere." All these stories and the **Feelings** that go along with them are merely obstacles and distractions to avoid dealing with life directly.

As with many people, my life story wasn't a pretty one. Much of my adult life has been spent pursuing various paths in search of **Freedom** from my past. Each of the paths was useful in some way and yet I continued to **Feel** stuck, haunted by my past story, **Feeling** unhappy, and trapped by something that was no longer real or true. Somehow, I was still a child living in my **Family** home and relating to my present life from that past place.

It wasn't until my husband died that I was confronted with having to live my life differently. I shifted from being an unconscious victim to a conscious player on the stage that is my life. The shock of my husband's death rocked me to the core of my being where I saw how unhappy I was and had always been. My opportunity had arrived; I knew it was now or never.

I spent two years in utter desolation and grief questioning my very existence ("soul searching," you might call it). With the help of a wonderful grief counsellor, I began to dig deep, to dismantle the false package I had constructed in order to live my life. I began to explore ways to live my life authentically. It was as though a veil began to lift and I could see from behind my cloud of sadness and despair. In time, I happened upon a Buddhist meditation course that piqued my interest. Little did I know that the journey I was about to embark upon would change my life.

Seven years later, with the help of my teacher (for whom I am deeply grateful) and my meditation practice, I am slowly developing an awareness of these many patterns as I work toward being able to interrupt them. My practice helps me to come into awareness, **Feel** the **Feelings** that arise, and be present in what is happening now, today, and not from the place of yesterday. Today I am able to **Feel** joy and moments of **Freedom** from my past. This new reality provides me with a renewed energy and alertness I have not experienced before. This success has informed me that it is possible for me to have even more of this new reality.

In the past, I often **Felt** like I was in a trance and not present. Today, I have learned that being awake is the path to living a **Full** life. That character, "it," has no interest in my being awake and present; "it" only wants to continue to keep me disconnected from the truth and asleep. At times my life work—my practice of staying present and aware—has been very difficult. In spite of that difficulty, I keep calm and carry on (although occasionally I have a tantrum or two). To move beyond myself through my practice and to be there for others in this present moment has become my passion. This new passion is the path that has given me both a voice to work with "it," and at the same time, a vehicle for self-care that has enabled me to change my life.

Korina is a client who has demonstrated such commitment to her own personal growth during our work together that I am regularly in awe of her "stick-with-it-ness."

Korina's Story

Why do some people seem to succeed so easily while others have difficulty reaching the simplest of goals? What holds us back from achieving greatness? Could it have something to do with that small, yet powerful, voice in the deepest part of us that has been a lifetime in the making? Is it the ghost of a voice from a parent, a sibling, a teacher, or a **Friend** trying to keep us safe, still, and possibly even controllable? These are some of the questions I ask myself as I consider where and how I'd like to move **Forward** with my life. How do I crawl out from under a lifetime of obeying, listening, and pleasing? It's a past that included behaviours that no longer serve me. I know that the voices driving those behaviours are no longer relevant. How will I gather the strength and the **Fortitude** to help me get to where I want to go? I know no one else can do it for me.

The **Fact** that I know I am not alone with this challenge brings me comfort; my questions and life experiences are not uncommon. I've accepted that life is a process of growth and I'm learning the value of treating myself with the same kindness and compassion I treat my children. This is the place where I started my journey; this premise is the stable **Foundation** that I use as my jumping-off point.

My goal was and still is to practise healthy self-care. My voyage along this path began years ago and just started to take momentum when I acquired a coach. It was a new experience that provided a new perspective. My coach helped me to *hear* myself. It was as though I was listening, maybe for the **First** time, to the person I was born to be, a person I had somehow lost sight of along the way. It was then, with the help of my coach, that I began to learn more about what I needed to do for myself and to come to a place where I truly believe that taking care of my own needs is my responsibility. The more self-aware and self-empowered I become, the better able I am to live a healthy happy life, a life where I **Feel** strong and ready to fulfill the role of wife, mother, daughter, sibling, **Friend**, and colleague. The further I move along this path of self-care the more distant those negative voices become.

They were still there though, at times, screaming things like, "Who do you think you are?" "How can you be so selfish?" The answer was simple, but not easy. I needed to be diligent and stick to my new practice of self-care because, when I didn't, I would slip back into the same old patterns that no longer served me, the behaviours that were comfortable and familiar, and that still held me captive. I no longer wanted to be held prisoner. I wanted to run and explore and be the best person I can be. I wanted to get to know myself better; I wanted to be a person whom I would call my best **Friend**.

Each day I improve my ability to be as good to myself as I am to others. Now in hindsight, I find it interesting that I had previously interpreted the saying, "Treat others as you would like to be treated" as "Look for ways to treat others better than the way you treat yourself." The kindness and patience I extended to my children are now the same I give myself. I laugh at my mistakes and celebrate my successes. During times of stress when that negative voice finds a way to say, "I told you so; go back to the way things used to be," I repeat a mantra quietly and softly to myself. "Everything will be fine, everything will work out. Everything will be fine, everything will work out." I repeat this until I am too tired to think of whatever had been bothering me and, as if by magic, in that exhaustion I am able to release it. The best part is that everything is fine and everything is working out.

Today I begin each morning by consciously and intentionally strategizing to give myself the gift of self-care, the care I would offer a newborn child who needs me more than anything else. I now know that if I don't care for myself, no one else will either. Through self-care, I can now see that I am lovable and I am loved. I deserve the best. I deserve to do, be, and have the best life possible.

My strategy of "Everything will be fine, everything will work out" (repeat until exhausted and wait for the results), helps me to make self-care a priority in my life. I remember this success and use it to manage that negative little voice whenever it makes an appearance in my life.

> *Jim is another colleague who is masterful in his ability to create a powerful visual image while at the same time keeping that visual simple and clean so it's easy to understand.*

Jim's Story

Sometimes I find myself in the hurricane of life, that place where it is swirling and confusing and gremlin-infested and **Full** of ego and, well, not happy. I need refuge. Where, in me, is there a place of refuge?

When I put the actual words of the gremlin in my hand and take the time to look at them by holding them at arm's length, I begin to gain some new perspective. If I also take the memory of those times in my life when I've been absolutely certain, when there was no shred of doubt in my decision, and place the words that describe those memories in my other hand I can become the

Observer. As an Observer, I am in a place of choice. When I do this, I put myself into the eye of the hurricane that I live in. It is totally calm here and I can see the two sets of words sitting in my hands. From this perspective, it is easier for me to see what is gremlin and what is truth. From this place of calm, I **Feel** more powerful and am able to tap into the objectivity that supports me in **Feeling** confident to act on a decision.

> *Courage and logic are two of the ingredients that Anne used in winning her battle against negative self-talk.*

Anne's Story

My story begins with my world being turned upside down by that "special someone" who had me believing I could leave everything behind and start anew. While the romance part was very easy—the starting anew wasn't.

My soul mate and I met while on vacation—I knew almost instantly he was the one I'd waited my entire life to meet. Initially, it was all so natural: the hurdles were tiny and easily overcome. The fear and self-doubt began a little later when the problems grew in size and we were faced with the **Full** force of reality and all the external factors that seemed determined to stop us from beginning a life together. Complications and barriers had their basis in the insurmountable **Facts** that we were citizens of different countries, that we were both **Fully** engaged in divorce proceedings, and that each of us had great careers and **Families** who depended on us at home.

Where would we live? Which of us would give up their career? What if his kids didn't accept me? What if they hate me? What will people say about my getting into another relationship when my divorce isn't even final? Would one of us resent the other if they moved and then couldn't restart their career? What are our options? Do I really, really love this person enough to take a chance and give up the life I've created for myself? Am I prepared to leave the country of my birth and all that that means?

These doubts made my head spin and as I look back I can see that some of these questions were logical and needed to be asked. Others were nothing more than fear-based. The internal dialogue I had to fight through to get to where I am today created a wild ride!

It is said that love conquers all, can it really? I had been advised by **Friends** that sometimes just being in love isn't enough and you need to be prepared for the reality of what you're getting into. It was good advice! I needed to work out a plan and then work to make it happen if I wanted to begin a life with this man of my dreams. "Plan the work and work the plan" was something I'd read somewhere—perhaps this was the time to put those words into action. Maybe this would be my key to success rather than just taking things as they came.

I knew I deserved to be happy and in love, and that was my goal. I knew I didn't want to be poor, and that was a goal. So what to do? "Plan the work and work the plan!" That day when I got really clear on those two goals was the same day I began to strategize with intention toward achieving them. It wasn't always easy and there were times that fear and self-doubt crept back into the process. By having a plan and the commitment to **Follow** it, along with the motivation of being able to see the process I was (we were) making in moving toward our goals, there was light at the end of the tunnel.

A logical approach and **Flexibility** were two of the key factors I used, both in creating my plan and in implementing it. I paid particular attention to how my choices would impact others. I gathered information and accessed resources regarding the legalities of emigrating to another country. I researched employment opportunities in my field and identified any further education that might be needed to accommodate the international nature of my pending move. I got clear on which battlefields I was prepared to die. That meant that I had to stay **Flexible** enough to be able to let go of my ego and walk away from issues that were getting in the way of my goals.

Change is hard, and at the same time change can be liberating in ways I never expected. I have had amazing opportunities because of my decision to "plan the work and work the plan" in pursuit of my goals. My life is **Full** of so many rewards now, including three wonderful grandchildren, something I never thought I would be **Fortunate** enough to have. I am a very lucky person and I truly believe we make our own luck. Perhaps luck is really about making the right decisions to move ahead and challenge the **Future** with a good "plan."

> *Maria's references to the physical release she Feels as she manages her negative self-talk caught my attention as they are quite different from anything else I'd heard until I received her submission. Perhaps you too will connect with her story in a new and different way.*

Maria's Story

My life is **Full** and wonderful! I work **Full** time, have two great children, and own my own business. Now for the "but"—I also have an unwelcome guest in my life. His name is Fred and he likes to run around in my head! Sometimes he causes a frenzy; sometimes he makes me freeze in place! He usually visits when there is a lot going on and is able to transform something that should have been "easy" into something that could not be more difficult.

When Fred arrives (and I actually notice him), I **First** take a break from what I am doing, stand up, stretch, and if I can, close my eyes. I am better able to ground myself with my eyes closed. My goal is to empty my mind and get into the present moment. This allows me space to stop worrying about what has happened in the past, or what might be coming in the **Future**. When I live in the past or the **Future**, Fred has way more power over my life. When I'm truly in the present, I can literally **Feel** him detaching from my head! Another strategy I use to get myself into the present is to go for a walk and really **Focus** on noticing what I see. This is about quieting my mind and again, paying attention to what I really need right now.

Something I've realized over the last year or so is that keeping Fred at bay is easier if I'm proactive. Recently I've added in a daily quiet time to my life (only ten minutes) where I don't do anything. I lie on the floor with my eyes closed and pay attention to each body part from my toe nails to the top of my head. Practising this seems to make it easier for me to manage everything in my life with much more success!

Now that I recognize Fred and have some strategies to keep him out of my head and in his place, I'm able to take clear action to stay on course and keep doing all the important things that I want to do in my life!

> *Jean's ability to create her powerful paradigm shift speaks for itself. Way to go, Jean!*

Jean's Story

Settling the little man on my shoulder wasn't as much about negative self-talk as it was about managing my fear during a life-changing experience with cancer. While negative self-talk and fear management may seem different at first glance, I suspect negative self-talk might be based in fear so maybe they're not so dissimilar after all.

I realized that I needed help so I asked for it. That was step one.

Step two came in the form of a course called "Managing Life with Cancer" through which I began to realize that my fear and worry were doing nothing other than causing me stress and grief. My learning in the course helped me to realize that we are all going to die one day. Once I was able to accept that, I was no longer living in fear of a return of the cancer. The course also helped me to find my new normal and new coping skills, which included relaxation techniques.

Step three was about managing the abundance of "talk" that was coming at me from outside sources. Others had a myriad of opinions about the cancer and many of them were negative. To manage these external influences I **Focused** on the realization that it was people projecting their fear onto me and it was not part of my journey.

Step four was really just a repeat of steps one, two, and three. Each time the cancer returned or a new one developed, I would ask for help, draw on those around me in my support network, deepen my learning of the new strategies that were helping me manage the fear, and shut out any external negativity that was trying to creep in.

Sometime in the last year, the little guy who had been jumping up and down on my shoulder started to sit more quietly. I am **Focused** on living rather than on dying, and taking each day as it comes.

CHAPTER
5

YOUR TURN

Earlier in this book, I promised you would have plenty of opportunity to pull out your pen and use this book as your own personal journal. This is the point where you really begin to make it your own. By customizing the pages of your book in this interactive way, you will develop your own personal guide.

Don't worry, there will be lots more to read too and I encourage you to take your time, to go through the pages and the stages one by one as you answer the questions for yourself. This book is private, it's yours, and no one will see it unless you choose to share it with them. Some of the questions will be more difficult than others. Do your best to answer them. You might choose to leave them till later when you've had some time to reflect on the questions and your responses. Or you may decide you want to go back and change what you've written. One little mantra that I like to use during times when I'm considering changing an answer is, "The best thing about a mind is that it can change." Somehow, those few little words seem to provide a new level of permission when I'm second-guessing myself. Having said that, I also encourage you to trust your initial instincts. Your responses are all right (meaning "they are all correct"). They're yours—they can't be anything other than right, as no one else could possibly know your truth.

Remember, there is no rush. This is you taking care of yourself. You picked up this book for a reason—you were interested in self-care and you were ready to move to action. Remember, self-awareness is step one in self-care and these questions are all about you, so pick up that pen and dive into the process of connecting with yourself. Stay **Focused** on keeping this **Fun**—it's all about getting you to a place where you'll connect with your self-care goal.

Now that you've read the stories of others—can you relate to any or all of them? How do those stories correspond with or affect your own story?

_____

_____

_____

_____

_____

How do you manage the negative influences that try to stop you from moving **Forward** toward your goal(s)? You may recognize this question from a few pages ago—go back and review what you wrote there. Has your response changed at all? If so, what caused that shift?

_____

_____

_____

_____

What do you do when there's an external barrier?

_____

_____

_____

_____

How do you manage the internal voice(s)?

_____

_____

_____

_____

Which are more difficult for you—the internal or external barriers? Why do you think that is?

_____

_____

_____

_____

Fear is often identified as a barrier. When has fear blocked your way?

_____

_____

_____

_____

How effective were you in managing that fear? What specifically did you do to mitigate it?

_____

_____

_____

_____

What might you do differently if you had that exact same scenario to do over again?

_____

_____

_____

_____

Sometimes, the fear of success is identified as a barrier. Can you think of a time when the fear of success got in the way of your moving **Forward**?

_____

_____

_____

_____

Being intentional about managing the fear and barriers that get in the way of **Forward** momentum is **Foundational** in self-care. What supports or strategies do you draw upon (both external and internal)?

_____

_____

_____

_____

How might the momentum built by moving **Forward** (even one tiny step) help you to keep **Focused** on achieving your goal(s)?

_____

_____

_____

_____

Think of three examples where you beat your own negativity and achieved your goals.

_____

_____

_____

_____

What common denominators did you employ in those successes?

_____

_____

_____

_____

How do you think choice factored into your successes?

_____

_____

_____

_____

How did your previous successes impact your choice of planning and **Following** through for future "mazes"?

_____

_____

_____

_____

How will you intentionally shift the **Focus** from "What don't I have?" to "What do I have?"?

_____

_____

_____

_____

_____

List other things you'd like to note about your ability to manage negative self-talk.

_____

_____

_____

_____

_____

"It is not the years in your life but the life in your years that counts."
Adlai Stevenson

CHAPTER
6

WHAT FEEDS ME?

Self-care strategies can be elusive and for each of us the answer to the question "What Feeds Me?" will be as unique and diverse as we are. The common denominators are that self-care is intentional, and it is the practice of regular activities that supports us in living a healthy life where there is balance and an overall sense of well-being. The activities might be physical, mental, spiritual, or work-related. Ultimately, they're yours to decide about and to act on.

Self-care is not selfish. It is a healthy practice and essential to our ability to care for those around us. If you've ever taken a **First Aid** course, you'll know that one of the **First** things the instructors teach is to "ensure no further danger" before you begin to help the victim. On an airplane, they direct us to put on our own oxygen masks before assisting anyone else. The same holds true for self-care in day-to-day life. If we don't look after ourselves (and keep a supply of "cookies" on hand), we'll be in no shape to do all the things we want to do with our **Families**, **Friends**, and colleagues.

Self-care is simply loving ourselves and taking the time to prove it. "Love yourself **First** and everything else falls into line" was a **Favourite** quote of the late, great Lucille Ball. Something I hear myself saying to clients is, "Don't say anything about yourself that you wouldn't say about your best **Friend**." Once you put self-care into that context, it begins to make a lot of sense.

Imagine you were counselling a girlfriend or better still your own daughter. Can you hear yourself saying something like, "If you don't love yourself, how can you expect anyone else to?" If we can be so wise in the counsel of others we care about; what gets in the way of our being as good to ourselves? Just as we can advise those we care about, others will also help us to gain perspective on our own circumstances. And just as we can't do it for others, no one else can do it for us. Self-care is our responsibility: at the same time as you're generous with your care for others remember to be as kind and as generous with yourself.

Self-care is both your right and your responsibility. How prepared are you to take it on? On a scale of 1-10 where 1 is very low and 10 is very high, how ready are you right now?

1   2   3   4   5   6   7   8   9   10

How do you **Feel** about your self-assessed ranking on this question?

_____

_____

_____

_____

_____

Whatever your answer, read on, this book is designed to create opportunities for self-reflection with the goal of building a reality that is consistent with your vision. You're in the process of building a solid **Foundation** for your cookie jar to sit upon.

We all have room for improvement on the self-care scale. Regardless of where I was yesterday or where I am today, I know that tomorrow is a new day and a new opportunity to improve my ranking. Another thing I keep in the back of my mind is that I only get one shot at this life—just one body—just one turn. If my car begins to break down as it ages or is involved in an accident and needs repair, I can just get a new one. Not so with myself—this is the only chance I get so I had better make the most of this life. I deserve to make the most of it. We all deserve to live our best lives. By being intentional in recognizing and acting on our self-care strategies, we are increasing our odds for success on that front—and no one can do it for us. Our life is our own masterpiece.

One of my **Favourite** self-care examples is a personal one, and over the course of this short story, there are so many instances of self-care that speak to me. I love any opportunity to relive it, so here goes.

Travel is one of my **Favourite** things to engage in and I do it as often as I can. This story takes place during a trip to Asia. I was travelling around Thailand with a group of **Friends** and the opportunity arose to visit a temple atop a mountain that was technically in Cambodia. It was a Cambodian temple and accessible only through Thailand, as international borders had been moved as a result of the most recent conflict in that region. Even more interesting was that this Cambodian temple housed a Hindu deity that I was interested in seeing firsthand. Even during my trip to India, I hadn't had the opportunity to view Shiva Lingam; it is rare to find a temple that features it, especially outside India. Shiva Lingam is a statue that is believed by many to represent the source of life in nature. Typically, it is formed from natural materials. Man-made lingams are commonly carved from wood or stone, and nature's versions are made from rock or even ice. Shiva Lingam is considered by many to be of significant importance to women in their spiritual practice.

Our bus made the journey to the end of the road, and the few of us who were prepared to make the long hot climb hopped on the little train that would take us the rest of the way into Cambodian territory. From the train terminus, it was a very hot walk up to the top of the mountain where the temple stood.

The temperature was in excess of a hundred degrees and the humidity was a hundred percent. I'd moved way past the feminine term of "glistening" and into full-blown sweating in no time. In spite of the heat and humidity, I found the views breathtaking. The Mekong River meandered its way through the jungles in the distance off to my left. There were children **Following** me up the mountain. While I was literally dragging myself up the hill, they were effortlessly hopping from rock to rock seeming not to **Feel** the heat or the climb at all.

I was carrying with me some traditional offerings of respect that I would leave in the temple sanctuary once I reached the top of the mountain. I had a lotus bud, some incense, and a few pieces of gold leaf.

Finally, we made it to the temple. My **Friends** who had made the climb with me opted to just peek in the temple doorway and then go to the edge of the mountaintop where they could enjoy the views. I'd climbed too far to settle for that though and so took my shoes off and entered the sacred space. Once inside the sanctuary I made my way to the base of Shiva Lingam where I lit my incense, rubbed my gold leaf onto the designated area, left my lotus bud, and had my moment of quiet reflection.

As I began to back out of the sanctuary, Tom, my guide who was sitting with the Thai Buddhist monk in residence, grabbed my hand and told me that the monk had invited me to stay as he would like to give me a blessing. What an honour! I immediately sat down on the mat beside Tom, and the monk proceeded to prepare for his blessing.

I wouldn't describe myself as a religious person; however, I am deeply spiritual and I respect the diversity that our world enjoys on this front. Being given the gift of a blessing from this Thai Buddhist monk in a Cambodian temple that housed a Hindu deity was like the coming together of the heart of so many cultures.

The monk used a bamboo brush that looked like a bunch of pick-up sticks bound together at one end. He dipped this brush into a big silver bowl of some kind of holy water and Tom instructed me to close my eyes. The monk proceeded to chant and sprinkle me with holy water for the next several minutes. I'm not certain just how long the blessing lasted, but it was definitely more than five minutes and probably closer to ten. Magically, that water he was spraying me with **Felt** like it had come out of a refrigerator and yet I knew that it hadn't. There was no power for miles around and the temperature outside was still over one hundred degrees. For me that cool water was like a miracle that revived my body and restored my soul. This was a powerful exercise in self-care that I will never forget. I had said "yes" to the opportunity, had chosen to take the time, had opened my heart and soul to receiving the gift, and had been able to stay present in the moment for the duration of the experience.

When the blessing was nearing completion, Tom instructed me to open my eyes and the monk finished his benediction by dipping his hand into the holy water and then making the sign of a cross on me. This final gesture appeared to me to be his attempt to incorporate some of what he would have believed to be my religious practice into his blessing. I was so moved by that gesture. If only the world could take a lesson from this Thai Buddhist monk who was able to see beyond the colour of my skin and the norms of my culture to a place where our differences were secondary and respect was the focus. His was an ultimate gesture of appreciation in these diverse circumstances. His willingness to adjust his blessing to accommodate one of my culture's commonly held religious practices was so pure and simple and yet so **Filled** with power and impact that I **Felt** something shift deep inside me and I knew I'd remember this experience **Forever**.

As I skipped back down the mountain **Feeling** like I was as young as the children around me, I knew I would be **Forever** changed by this experience. Travel itself is part of my self-care practice; speaking up and saying that I wanted to go visit this temple was another example of self-care; taking the time with my offering and choosing to say yes to receive the blessing were also examples of putting my self-care practice into action.

Although it would be easy for me to end my story here, I will continue just a little further and tell you that the magical momentum of this day filled with self-care continued even longer. Because I had spent so much time in the sanctuary on the mountaintop, my **Friends** had all made the journey back down before me: I was the last to leave. At the bottom of the mountain, I got back on the final train of the day to make the return trip into Thailand where I would reconnect with my **Friends** .

Once back with my group, I discovered that someone had ordered lunch for me already so it was waiting for me as soon as I arrived. What a bonus! Surely, it couldn't get any better than this—and yet it did.

After lunch, a **Friend** and I were walking through the market area of this little mountain village when I **Felt** two skinny arms wrap around my waist from the back. I could hear the giggling and knew immediately that this hug was coming from a local Thai resident. When I finally got the hugger to show her face, I discovered a wizened little woman who had a smile that reached from ear to ear and who was obviously very excited to be able to give me a hug.

I stand out in places like Asia. I am white skinned, I have blonde hair, blue eyes, and I have a large frame so I look very different from anyone who lives there and even from the typical tourist who visits remote areas such as this region. This little woman was giving me a hug that was filled with all the excitement you might imagine would come from a small child who had just received a gift they'd been dreaming about. In that moment I realized that as much as I had just seen and experienced a life-changing event in the temple on top of the mountain so had she. I represented her cultural adventure—an international memory that had come to her on her home ground. It was explained to me that she had heard about people who looked like me but never thought she would actually see one!

Yes—this is a memory that I draw on often. It truly was a day when I stayed completely present and lived **Fully** in the moment. It was a day when I was completely committed to saying "yes" to myself and a time when I was able to experience the magic of both giving and receiving.

Not all my stories are packed with self-care.

I recall another day that was not nearly as **Filled** with smiles and joy and that was equally memorable. It continues to provide me with a touchstone on what can happen when the busyness of life opens the door to neglect on the self-care front. It was during a time when my life was ripe with great excuses not to practise regular self-care. I was married, with two busy and rapidly growing children, working full time, volunteering on several committees, and still trying to be a super mom on the home front too.

The month was August and the summer's bounty was abundant. Blueberries were hanging on the berry bushes and my **Family** had been begging for a blueberry pie for weeks. In hindsight, there are a million things I could have done differently. And as we've already established, looking at anything from the endpoint makes the picture a whole lot clearer than it is when you're in the midst of it.

It was the weekend after a long and busy workweek. Saturday and Sunday were the days when I got everything done in the home: housework, shopping, cooking for the week, laundry—the list was endless. This weekend was likely the end of the blueberry harvest and so if I was going to do it, it had to be now or never. This would probably be my last chance till this same time next year.

Did I run to the store to pick up a pre-made crust you wonder? Of course not—I was a super mom and could do anything and everything! Here's an overview of what transpired inside my head over the next couple of hours. It's a look at the thoughts that were running through my mind so you can get a sense of the story from my perspective in that moment on that day during that time in my life. It was a busy time and I'm pretty sure my thinking speed and my productivity was running in overdrive!

Cut the shortening into the flour.
Remind the kids to get their homework finished.
Add just enough ice water to get the dough to come together without becoming tough.
Ask the husband to turn down the TV.
Be careful not to overwork the dough!
Let the dog out.
Roll the pastry into perfect circles and put it in the pie plate. Don't forget to preheat the oven. Mix the blueberries, sugar, and tapioca and pour into the bottom crust.
Let the dog back into the house.
Roll out the top crust and fold it into quarters. Make little cuts in the dough so the steam will be able to escape while the pie is baking. Damn! Forgot to lower the oven rack to lowest position before turning it on so get out oven mitts and do it now. Place the top crust onto the pie and sprinkle with a little extra sugar and cinnamon. Put the pie onto the bottom rack for fifteen minutes.
Boy, this looks like a really good pie!
Get supper underway. It will be a traditional meal of meatloaf, potatoes, and vegetables tonight. The oven is already on and that menu will go well with the pie.
It will be just like Grandma used to make. Wonder if Grandma ever got tired. Wonder if life really was simpler back then, in Grandma's day.

Hopefully, there will be leftovers for lunches during the week. Meatloaf sandwiches—can't remember the last time I had one of those.

Let the dog out again.

Check that the kids are still doing their homework.

Eeek! Turn the oven down so the pie can finish baking and the crust doesn't burn.

Put the potatoes and vegetables on to cook.

Go look at whatever it is that the husband wants me to see on TV.

Let the dog back inside.

Check the potatoes. Yes, they're finished and there is still time to mash them as that is a Family Favourite. Veggies are finished too. Perfect timing.

I really can do it all!

Save the potato and vegetable water to add to the pot of soup I'm making after dinner tonight so we'll have it for dinner sometime during the week. I can make biscuits to go with the soup. Gads, don't worry about that now—that's another day!

Why don't I have more counter space? What are all these papers piled on the counter taking up the space I need? Oops—forgot about those bills to be paid. After dinner, I'll get to them.

Potatoes are mashed, meatloaf is resting on the counter, pie is done, and it's ready to come out of the oven. Wow! I'm hot! Where will I put this pie to cool? Sigh—I'll just put it on the back burner of the stove. That way it won't get bumped in the rush to get food onto plates and no one will be burned by the hot pie plate. It's also a perfect spot as there is absolutely not an inch of space left on the counter!

This might be the best-looking pie I've ever baked! If it tastes half as good as it looks, I am a super mom!

Remind the kids that the pie is too hot just yet and they need to have their supper and let it cool before they dive into it.

The house smells amazing. Feeling super proud of my accomplishment.

Remind myself that I'm not done yet. Dishes to do. Bills to pay. Laundry still in the washer.

Dog wants out again.

Sit down at the table to enjoy this amazing dinner.

Thinking about that piece of fresh blueberry pie I'm going to have after dinner. Might even put a scoop of ice cream on it. Can picture the ice cream melting over the still "warm from the oven" pie. Doesn't get any fresher than that. Pastry from scratch, freshly picked blueberries, pie handmade with love.

Focus on the dinner first!

Find out about how school was during the week. Don't often have much time to talk to the kids about how things are going.

Finally starting to relax.

Someone else can let the dog in this time.

This dinner really is delicious. I think I might have outdone myself tonight and the pie is still to come. Everyone looks so happy and they're all enjoying dinner together. What a rare treat.

And that's when it happened. There was the combined sound of broken glass and an explosion. We all ran into the kitchen to discover that my beautiful magazine-cover-quality pie had literally exploded. There were blueberries everywhere. I wanted to cry. I didn't know what to do or how this could have happened. It took a minute before I could figure it out. In my haste and multitasking, I had neglected to turn off the burner that I had set the pie on to cool. Pyrex® pie plates are not intended for stovetop use and this was the result. Glass and blueberries everywhere and no pie for any of us.

It was a sad day and a memory that I reflect on when I think of the times in my life when my self-care practices were lacking.

Each of us measures our self-care strategies differently. My story about the temple atop a mountain will make sense to some of you and others might find more common ground in my story about the pie. Or perhaps this next example of intentional attention and commitment to self-care that Steve Jobs brings to light in this recap of a speech he made will be a match for the rest of you.

During an address to a graduating class at Stanford in June 2005, Steve Jobs, CEO of Apple Computers and Pixar Animation Studios, recalled a quote that had resonated for him. That quote went something like this: "If you live each day as if it were your last, someday you will be right." He continued by describing how from that day forward he made it a point to look in the mirror every morning so he could ask himself an intentional question. His question was to consider whether, if this were the last day of his life, he would want to do what he had planned to do for the day. In his speech he concluded by explaining that if his answer was "no" for too many days in a row, it would be a sign that something needed to change (Stanford University 2005).

Did Steve Jobs understand self-care? Was he able to implement a strategy that enabled him to stay connected to his goals, his dreams, and his passion? For me, his address sums up a strategy he used to help keep his cookie jar **Full**.

Sadly though, not everyone keeps their cookie jar **Full**. Self-care eludes them and for whatever reason they never tap into the ready supply of opportunities they could use to **Fill** their jar. Examples of this are everywhere. Look around at the people you know. Some of them are taking big bites out of life and living every moment to its **Fullest**. Others aren't. Which path do you **Follow**? My preference is to take big bites and live life juicily.

Here is a little bite out of one woman's story. She chose to **Follow** the empty jar path. It's a true story—a story I describe as one of the saddest I've ever shared. It's a story that helps motivate me to stay on the path to keeping my jar **Full**. It's one that influences me to subscribe to Steve Jobs' model of checking in daily to make sure I'm on track and living my life in a way that is consistent with my passion, my values, and my interests.

I heard this unhappy account while visiting a **Friend** who had recently celebrated her sixty-first birthday and who was now in the final stages of her life. Cancer had taken its toll and she had moved into hospice care. During the visit, my **Friend** said something that I'll never forget. With sadness in her voice and tears in her eyes she said, "I missed my turn." Those four little words spoke volumes—she had wanted to travel, to uncover adventures, to write a book, to get a motorhome and explore North America, and to spend more time with her **Family** and **Friends**. Instead, she had chosen a life in which she was chained to her desk, waiting, always waiting for the day she would retire, the day she would be able to do all the things she dreamt about. Retirement never came for her. She died before that happened.

For me, the learning in this story is not in her words, "I missed my turn"; it is in her unspoken words—the reframed meaning of those words—what she meant to say in hindsight, "I didn't like the turn I took." I will **Forever** be grateful to my **Friend** for this life lesson and I am very proud of myself for having chosen to learn from it.

How will you choose to apply the learning from this story in your life?

_____

_____

_____

_____

_____

These past few pages really are the **Foundation** of how I practise self-care. I remind myself to check in every day to see if I'm on track, whether I have a clear understanding of the things that **Feed** me and the things that don't. I use the worst case scenario (my dying **Friend's** story) as a means to stay motivated and on track, and I work to stay **Focused** on the present, because what is past is past, and what will be will be, regardless of whether or not I worry about it. Specifics that **Feed** me and **Fill** my cookie jar include cuddling with my grandkids, spending time with my adult children, exploring exotic lands and appreciating the cultural experiences they offer, giggling with girlfriends, having **Fun** with **Family**, watching a movie that makes me cry or a movie that makes me laugh, taking a long hot shower, lying in a hammock, reading a great book, and taking time for meditation and reflection. The list could go on for pages: **Fresh** air, the wind, the smell of cinnamon buns straight from the oven …. They all stimulate my senses and often evoke memories. I can conjure them up in my mind's eye and each time I enjoy one of these "cookies" that represent my self-care strategies, I recognize it for what it is—self-care. I consciously put it in my cookie jar and pay attention to just how **Full** (or empty) my jar is.

What kinds of things does your cookie list include?

_____

_____

_____

_____

_____

"If you don't like the road you're walking, start paving another one."
Dolly Parton

CHAPTER
7

STOP THE WORLD; I WANT TO GET OFF!

Life can be tough some days and committing to a regular and intentional self-care practice is not always easy. On the days that I hear myself say anything that even remotely resembles the obvious sign of imbalance that this chapter title suggests, I am thrown into a time warp. It's an age when I revisit the memory of an image that created such an impression on my young mind that it stuck with me to this day. It's an image that was simultaneously disturbing and hilarious, and that evoked enough of an emotional response from me that it is **Forever** imprinted on my memory. It's not really a bad picture, just a picture that was bizarre enough to become the visual that flashes before me any time I **Feel** overwhelmed by life. But … before I share the image with you I'd like to set the stage and give you some context so please bear with me as I close my eyes and go back to the day that I first saw it.

An anecdotal equation for you to consider as I prepare to tell my story. Young minds are such curious things + fads that come and go through the ages = an example of what can form our lifelong <u>Filters</u> .

It was the early 1960s, a simpler time. There were no video games and even television was a rare treat. Man had not yet landed on the moon and I was about six or seven years old—not worldly at all. Although I don't remember the specifics, I recall that my **Family** was spending the day with **Friends** we'd never visited before. I was shy, impressionable, and awed by the decor, the stories, and the many differences that our hosts' home presented. Somehow their place seemed a little more exotic, a little more colourful, and maybe even a little dangerous in comparison to the haven that was my childhood home. My younger sister and I were excited at the prospect of spending the day exploring and discovering the treasures their home had to offer. There was adventure in the opportunity. Kids were easily occupied in those days.

We examined all the photos in the living room, considered the **Fancy** cushions on the sofa, and enjoyed a cookie and a glass of milk with the grown-ups at the kitchen table. We played with the toys provided and coloured in the colouring books we had brought along to keep us busy.

It wasn't long before I had to visit the bathroom and that is where I discovered the image that would become a visual tool I've reflected on for the rest of my life. A 1960s bathroom didn't conjure up the spa-like tranquility of the restrooms of today—they were more likely filled with knick-knacks, crocheted doilies, and knitted toilet paper and tissue box covers. This particular bathroom also sported a **Fancy** fabric cover for the lid of the toilet seat, and when I saw the picture on that fabric cover I almost forgot why I'd come into the bathroom in the **First** place! There on the lid of the toilet was an illustration of a man inside the toilet bowl. Just his head and shoulders were above the seat. He was reaching up to pull the chain that would flush him down the drain and the look on his face was one of desperation. The caption beneath the picture read, "Goodbye, cruel world!"

My hope is that this image has given you cause to chuckle or smile as that is my reaction to the memory today. The reason I share it with you now is to offer perspective on the insanity and imbalance our world seems to accept as normal. Practising healthy self-care requires perspective, commitment, and balance in all areas of our lives. Perspective provides clarity, commitment helps us to **Follow** through, and balance is the scale that supports **Fair** and equitable shares for all the compartments that make up our life.

"Balance" is a word that resonates for me and the one that I use as a "go to" in my self-care practice. The image that comes with this childhood memory helps me to move back toward a healthier position, when the external (and sometimes internal) forces of life become too much.

What are some of the interesting memories you recall from your youth?

How do they impact the choices you make today?

_____

_____

_____

_____

_____

CHAPTER
8

DON'T SHOULD ON YOURSELF

The play on words here is intentional. Just as you ought not defecate on yourself—should-ing is not much better. Occasionally when coaching a client, I will hear them use the word *should* while they describe an issue or goal they're **Focused** on. That word is a clue for me to gather more information so my client can hear themselves explore their motivation, attachment, and expectations that may be connected to the sacrifice that is the thing they say they *should* do.

Should can get in the way of so many things and it can be a great place to hide too. The problem with using it as a hiding place or allowing it to be a barrier to moving in a direction we want to go is that it really can keep us at a standstill for a very long time. Hiding behind *should* is more common than you might think. On this topic, I recall one client I was working with in particular. She was very skilled at hiding behind *should*. The day I remember though is the day that she stopped hiding behind it—the day that she had her epiphany—the day that she decided hiding behind *should* was no longer serving her.

This particular client was very **Fond** of describing how much she disliked her work. She really was a glass-half-empty type of person. She often talked about how she should have pursued her dream of becoming a lawyer and regularly retold the stories of what had gotten in the way of her career goals and aspirations.

It was during one of our meetings that happened to coincide with her fiftieth birthday. Again, she was choosing to see herself as a victim in her life—a person who was destined to live out the rest of her years in a job she "hated."

As she regaled me with her woes and the lost option of becoming a lawyer, I asked her how long it takes to become a lawyer. She replied that she had checked into it once and was told that it would take her a **Full** seven years—a long and impossible commitment at her age. I asked her how old she would be at graduation if she were to start today and she replied, "Fifty-seven."

I was quiet for a minute and then I said, "You're going to be fifty-seven anyway, so you might as well be a fifty-seven-year-old lawyer." It was as though she'd never considered that angle before and after a few moments of deafening silence she nodded her head and said, "You're right; I could." That was the day that she moved from hiding behind *should* and began using the hope that lives in *could* to propel her **Forward** in the direction of her goal.

That same client just celebrated her fifty-fifth birthday and she will begin articling next year. She is very excited and loves the **Fact** that she has not only survived, she has in fact, thrived in the educational experience. She is *soooo* close to her goal now that she can actually taste it and the last time we met, all of her *shoulds* had turned into *coulds, haves,* and *wills.*

Should can often get in the way of healthy self-care so I encourage you to listen carefully and when you hear yourself use that word, consider questions that will help you get in touch with your own motivation and attachment to outcomes. Is this *should* based in sacrifice that has an expectation of reciprocity attached to it? If so, how healthy does that **Feel**? Is this *should* obligatory or is it something you really want to do? Getting clear on the motivation to do something can make the sense of accomplishment at the end of the doing that much sweeter.

If your *should* is prompted by sacrifice, you have moved into the realm of sacrifice and expectation, and I believe that is a no-win game. In my experience, every sacrifice has an expectation attached to it. We may not see it at **First** glance; however, I believe the expectation is there.

Imagine you're travelling with a **Friend** who wants to do something you don't want to do. You say "no" and yet the **Friend** pleads with you to go along as they're uncomfortable going on their own. At that point, you get to decide—you can choose to stick with your "no" and in a mutually beneficial relationship, your choice will be respected. If you change your answer to "yes" because you **Feel** you *should*, you've entered the game; and I believe the next time you want your **Friend** to do something that they don't want to do, you will think that they *should* (an expectation). However, if you say "yes" because it's more important to you that your **Friend Feel** supported in what they want to experience than it is for you to not go, you will have made a choice. Choice is the opposite of sacrifice and choice overrides *should* every time. All expectation leads to is a high potential for disappointment.

Perhaps the **Fact** that the word "should" and the word "shovel" both begin with "sh" is no accident. Maybe "should" is a quiet (shhh) code that triggers us to use our questions and curiosity as shovels to dig deeper and uncover a place where we take care of ourselves at the same time as we take care of obligations. In this place, curiosity leads to clarity and we move to action, not because we should, rather because we choose to.

Occasionally that *should* comes in the form of something you wish you had done in hindsight. In those cases, *should* becomes an easy excuse for a missed opportunity, much like the client who wished she'd gone to law school. In her case, she was able to dial in for clarity about what she really wanted by shifting her **Focus** to a **Forward** direction and in so doing she changed her life trajectory to one that she **Felt** good about. **Focusing** on what is already past versus what's in **Front** is also a no-win game.

My personal stance on this "shoulda, woulda, coulda" mantra may sound a little like tough love. I believe that if you think you should have done something, then you would have done it. That time is now past. **Forgive** yourself, learn from the experience, and move **Forward**. Next time, do it because you choose to.

"Twenty years from now you will be more disappointed by the things that you didn't do than by the ones you did do. So throw off the bowlines. Sail away from the safe harbour. Catch the trade winds in your sails. Explore. Dream. Discover."
Mark Twain

CHAPTER
9

GUYS NEED SELF-CARE TOO

While I admit this book was written with women in mind, I'd be remiss not to address the **Fact** that everyone deserves to have a plan for self-care. Some of us may be more willing or ready to admit our need for improved self-care than others are. When we just jump to the bottom line, we can see that we are all at risk if our cookie jar is empty. I write from a female perspective and the cookie jar analogy may not resonate for the men in your life. If you've got guys in your world, or if you're a guy reading this book, consider what makes sense from the male perspective. Women may be surprised just how insightful and skilled men are when it comes to practising self-care. Perhaps there are lessons we women can learn by **Following** their lead. My suspicion is that we women will find value in the learning and information we get from those conversations too.

During my research for this book, I had occasion to meet with several men on the topic of self-care. The real aha! I discovered during my interviews with them was how clear and capable they are of identifying what motivates them to incorporate self-care practices into their life and what they view as triggers in recognizing an "empty cookie jar."

In a nutshell, and this is very much a generalization, at their core, men believe they deserve to practise self-care. In **Fact**, they don't even refer to it as self-care: they call it "taking time for themselves to do what they want." I love men! They are so comfortable with saying it like it is. They know how to keep it simple and they are action-oriented. They don't think about it for so long that they miss opportunities and they are clear on what it is that they enjoy doing.

The real surprise for me, or maybe it wasn't as surprising as it was insightful, was that men don't view the symptoms of an empty jar as being attached to an emotional void. They actually refer to it as broken, physically broken. They talk about how, when they hit that wall, they notice that their physical body begins to break down. Their blood pressure goes up, their performance in the gym goes down, their cholesterol goes wonky, and … well, you get the picture. Either way, they recognize that they're being pulled in too many directions and that the pressures of their busy lives need to be balanced out with healthy self-care practices.

What is your reaction to my comments in this chapter?

_____

_____

_____

_____

_____

How will you apply this insight to your day-to-day life?

_____

_____

_____

_____

_____

Who, if anyone, would you like to have a conversation with about how they measure their own self-care?

_____

_____

_____

_____

_____

What will you ask them?

_____

_____

_____

_____

_____

When will you initiate that conversation?

_____

_____

_____

_____

"When the well is dry, we know the worth of water."
Benjamin Franklin

CHAPTER
10

FILL UP ON LIFE!

When we're exhausted by the demands and pressures of life, it can be really hard to stay connected or even aware of our passion. Finding ways to keep that cookie jar intact, so you can **Focus** on **Filling** it, are paramount. Here are a few quotes that demonstrate what some famous folk share as philosophies that help them stay on track.

- SARK (Susan Ariel Rainbow Kennedy) **Fills** up on life with beliefs such as, "Live Juicy" and "Plant impossible gardens."
- Howard Schultz of Starbucks has been known to recognize that his business success is at least in part because the company sees its customers as whole people. As a result everyone at Starbucks **Focuses** on **Filling** souls, not just bellies.
- "The best way to cheer yourself up is to try to cheer somebody else up" is Mark Twain's recipe for moving toward a **Full** life.
- The work of best-selling author and screenwriter Ayn Rand supports her personal interest in individualism and capitalism. Her commitment to live life on her own terms is reflected

in this quote from her novel *Atlas Shrugged*. "I swear—by my life and my love of it—that I will never live for another man, nor ask another man to live for mine."

- Martin Seligman, famed positive psychology author and professor, was able to prove his belief that living a meaningful life is the **Foundation** of happiness: he had his students compare the lasting effects between engaging in **Fun** activities and practising altruism through the doing of good deeds for others.
- Colin Powell believes that, "Perpetual optimism is a force multiplier."
- Winston Churchill said, "The pessimist sees difficulty in every opportunity and the optimist sees opportunity in every difficulty."
- Eckhart Tolle's message to the world and his own philosophy in life is, "It's always now."[1]
- And my personal **Favourite** is a message that Dr. Seuss shares in his best-selling book, *Oh, The Places You'll Go!* He reminds me that I have brains in my head and feet in my shoes so I get to steer myself in any direction I choose.

Where we've been in life does not determine where we will go. While we only get one shot at living our life, each day we have an opportunity for a fresh start. Creating our own personal story is a choice, so take a deep breath, pick up that pen, and consider these questions. Keep in mind that you are in control of this process. You have the power to give yourself permission to take a break at any time. Some of these questions will take time to consider so create some uninterrupted time and space for yourself so you will be able to **Focus**. You're worth it!

---

[1]From the book *Stillness Speaks*. Copyright © 2003 by Eckhart Tolle. Reprinted with permission of New World Library, Novato, CA. www.newworldlibrary.com

What would others say are your philosophies of life?

_____

_____

_____

_____

_____

What would some of your most notable quotes be?

_____

_____

_____

_____

_____

REALLY GOOD "F" WORDS

Are you happy with what they say? If not, how would you prefer to be remembered?

_____

_____

_____

_____

What can you do to create a bridge between how you're currently being quoted and how you'd like to be quoted?

_____

_____

_____

_____

What's stopping you from starting work on that today?

_____

_____

_____

_____

What is the **First** thing you will do to create that bridge?

_____

_____

_____

_____

When will you do that?

_____

_____

_____

_____

How will you hold yourself accountable to **Following** through on this plan?

_____

_____

_____

_____

CHAPTER
11

THREE FINGERS

While three fingers could have been a measure of whiskey just a few decades ago, in this context it refers to the three fingers that are pointing back at you every time you point your finger at another person. Try it for yourself: make a fist, stretch your arm out in **Front** of you, and then point at an object with your **First** finger as though you were pointing at another person. Hold that position and take a close look at your hand. Notice that there is just one finger pointing at the object and that there are three other fingers pointing back at you. In mathematical terms, those three fingers are like being pointed at to the third power!

It's always so much easier to see and know what others need to do to fix their situation. Whenever I hear myself advising another person on what they need to do, I visualize my hand and those three fingers that are pointing back at me. This three-finger rule is my reminder to ask myself, "What is it that I most need to hear right now?" How can I bring this advice I'm so intent on giving to another back to myself and apply it to whatever is going on in my life? What do I need to do to be able to hear myself?

Consider these questions as you explore your own relationship with the three-finger rule. How often do I hear myself advising others?

_____

_____

_____

_____

When I receive advice from others, how do I respond?

_____

_____

_____

_____

How does that differ from when I come to my own conclusions about next steps?

_____

_____

_____

_____

How will my responses to these last few questions affect me as I go **Forward** in life?

_____

_____

_____

_____

What will I do differently as a result?

_____

_____

_____

_____

I know I've **Felt** supported to come to my own conclusions about next steps at times. Why was that?

_____

_____

_____

_____

These were the things that encouraged and supported me to come to my own conclusions:

_____

_____

_____

_____

This differs from times when I've allowed others to influence my decision in the **Following** ways:

_____

_____

_____

_____

Which way is easier or more difficult: when I come to my own conclusions or when I allow others to influence my decisions?

_____

_____

_____

_____

What makes one way easier?

_____

_____

_____

_____

Which way takes longer?

_____

_____

_____

_____

_____

How does the amount of time required factor into my decision about which way to proceed?

_____

_____

_____

_____

Which style more closely matches the way I tend to behave in my support of others?

_____

_____

_____

_____

_____

What do I most like about the way I bring support to others?

_____

_____

_____

_____

What, if anything, will I do differently the next time I find myself on either the giving or the receiving end of a three-finger kind of circumstance?

_____

_____

_____

_____

_____

"If one advances confidently in the direction of one's dreams, and endeavors to live the life which one has imagined, one will meet with a success unexpected in common hours."
Henry David Thoreau

CHAPTER
12

MY FAVOURITE F WORDS

"**Friends, Fun, Forward**," and "**Focused**" are some of my **Favourite F** words. When you befriend them, they will be the cornerstone in building, maintaining, and getting what you want from your community of support. None of us can do it alone. Practising self-care creates a great opportunity to look around you for people and places that will lend their encouragement and assistance. It's also a chance for you to lend your backing to others in return. Giving can be one of the most satisfying and rewarding self-care strategies there are.

This chapter is dedicated to expanding your circle. Here is where you'll begin to pull together your own plan of action. A plan that suits your personality and interests. This chapter is the place where you'll take responsibility for initiating the processes that will support the action for creating and recognizing your own self-care.

Whether your preference is for technology or good old pen and paper, the time has come to identify the people you'd like to invite into your circle, your community of support. Think about it as your Cookie Jar Club, your Collection of Kindred Spirits, your Gathering of Good **Friends**, or any other name that captures *your* vision for *your* community of support. Keep it **Fun, Friendly,** and **Focused**—remember it is all about people, places, and activities that will support each other's common goal of self-care.

It's time to begin designing your customized action plan. We'll work through it one step at a time and before you know it, you'll be well on your way.

The first of my **Favourite F** words that we'll **Focus** on is "**Friends**." The number of **Friends** in your group is entirely up to you. My experience has taught me that fewer than three is too small and greater than ten is too large. Communities or networks of support may look very different for each of us. During my research for writing this book, I discovered that some interviewees describe their networks of support as **Faith**-based, while others say theirs has a cultural **Foundation**. Some describe them as having a common denominator of long-term **Friendship** and community at the core, and still others say they choose to subscribe to structured support groups that are driven by an external agenda. Regardless, they all provide the same thing—a safe environment where respect and common goals drive the direction and action.

Ask yourself these questions and take your time. There is no rush. Finding the right mix of **Friends, Fun,** and **Focus** is paramount.

Friends

What are some of the qualities I'm looking for in the **Friends** I invite into my community of support? (Examples might be "good listener, willing to share, reliable," etc.)

_____

_____

_____

_____

Who are some of the **Friends** I'd like to invite? (You know who they are.)

_____

_____

_____

_____

How will I prioritize this list so the group doesn't become too large, which might risk losing sight of our common goal? (If this is difficult, stay **Focused** on the desired outcome and refer back to the qualities you're looking for in the people you invite.)

_____

_____

_____

_____

How could we make sure these gatherings don't become a burden?

_____

_____

_____

_____

What signs or symptoms might appear to let us know our get-togethers are becoming burdensome or ineffective? (Examples might be "People have stopped attending." "It doesn't **Feel Fun.**")

_____

_____

_____

_____

Do we have to meet in person or could I include technology in creating a community of support? A social media group? (The sky or "the cloud" is the limit.)

_____

_____

_____

_____

Fun

Now it's time to move to the next **F—Fun**.
How do I know when I'm having **Fun**? (Examples might be: "I don't want to leave." "I laugh till I get a side ache." "I can hardly wait till I get to do it again.")

_____

_____

_____

_____

Events or activities that I've had **Fun** at in the past include these examples:

_____

_____

_____

_____

This is what made these events and activities **Fun**:

_____

_____

_____

_____

Who were some of the people at my **Fun** events? Recognizing this, do I need to go back to the previous page to add to or delete from the list of people I want to invite?

_____

_____

_____

_____

Events or activities from the past that have NOT been **Fun**:

_____

_____

_____

_____

Some reasons those activities or events weren't **Fun**:

_____

_____

_____

_____

How might I intentionally avoid some of these potential pitfalls?

_____

_____

_____

_____

Forward

Forward is another really good **F** word. By keeping an eye on the **Future** without losing our **Focus** on the present, and instead of regaling about the past, we spend our time on things we really can affect. The past is the past, and certainly the learning and experience we bring from that past helps make us who we are today. It doesn't dictate where we go from here though. By maintaining a **Forward** momentum in all that you do, you'll be spending your time on decisions and plans that you actually have a say in. It's easy to slip backward so don't go there. It's old news and may not be worth the time it takes to review it.

On a scale of 1 to 10, where 1 is not often and 10 is very often, how often do I stay **Forward Focused**? Circle your answer.

1   2   3   4   5   6   7   8   9   10

How do I **Feel** about this self-assessed ranking?

_____

_____

_____

_____

What, if anything, am I willing to do to change that score so it is closer to where I'd like it to be?

_____

_____

_____

_____

What gets in the way of my looking **Forward**?

_____

_____

_____

_____

How does it serve me to keep going back to the past? (Ask yourself this if it is something you find that you are prone to do.)

_____

_____

_____

_____

_____

If going back to the past doesn't serve me, what do I need to do to look **Forward** instead?

_____

_____

_____

_____

Focus

Now for the final **F** in this list of four **Foundational F** words—**Focus**. For the purpose of this exercise, we'll apply our **Focus** to the conversations we will have with others in the community of support we're building. Keep in mind it is your willingness to **Focus** that is the key. The ideas for this **F** will evolve and grow over time. Making an effort to get clear on your intention right from the outset will help you as you move **Forward**. When you're clearly able to describe an outcome, the odds of achieving it go up exponentially!

What do I want to get out of our gatherings? (Examples might be "**Fun** and **Friendship**"; "a **Feeling** of time well spent"; "ideas for our next get-together"; "a sense of camaraderie"; etc.)

_____

_____

_____

_____

_____

How will I know if at least some of my expectations have been met?

_____

_____

_____

_____

_____

What are my top three expectations in terms of outcomes for the group?

_____

_____

_____

_____

_____

Now that you've decided on whom you'd like to include in your community of support, it's time to make it official by inviting them to participate. This is where the work you've done over the past few pages will be really helpful. Those insights will be the material you'll be able to draw on as you answer the five W's (who, what, when, where, and why) in the process of designing your invitation.

Some of you may choose to invite your **Friends** via a digital invitation (there are lots of ideas to choose from online), create a social media event, or pick up the phone. There will be a few of you who love artistic activities so you will choose to use this as an opportunity to practise some self-care by pulling out all your crafting supplies and creating custom invitations from scratch. Whichever way you decide to move **Forward**—make it work for you. Be intentional in all your choices. If it doesn't support your goal of self-care, don't do it! Listen to your inner voice—if there is a *should* anywhere in there go back and reread chapter eight.

In your invitation, you will want to encourage everyone to get a copy of this book for themselves. You've been exploring your own level of readiness for self-care as you've worked through these pages, and it is only **Fair** that everyone come to the **First** gathering having had the same opportunity for self-awareness and **Familiarity** with the terminology and concepts they'll be using in the activities and conversations this book has designed for your gatherings.

Once everything is in place and you've begun the action of intentional self-care with your new group you'll notice that a special bond will develop as your community settles over time. The unique culture of your group will have its own rituals, norms, taboos, and beliefs. Take the time to explore them. As your group begins to take form, have a **Focused** group discussion about the possible changes that may occur as a group member leaves or a new person enters the picture. Google "stages of group development" and talk about forming, storming, norming, and performing.

As your group is in its very early stages of development, you may have to draw on past personal experience to come up with examples from other groups. Make plans for how your new group might recognize and learn the early phases of group development as they occur. Keep in mind that all stages of group development serve a purpose. Some of them may Feel more productive than others, but all are important and offer valuable lessons.

By spending a little time and effort to understand your unique customized community of support in the early stages, your network will be well positioned to be powerfully successful and filled with **Fun**!

Do take the time to do your own research. Here is a peek at the way I describe the stages. The word that identifies each of the stages is pretty self-explanatory in that first your group will come together (forming) and then there will be some rocky bits to traverse as you get to know one another (storming). At the same time, you'll begin building the rules of group engagement (norming) as you continue along the path to a place where your group shifts into the performing phase. It is very likely that groups will dance between the storming, norming, and performing stages during their lifetime, so don't despair if you see signs of that in your group —it's actually a sign of a healthy group because it means you're not stagnant.

P.S.

Even though I said I had just four <u>Favourite Foundational F</u> words—I'm going to add a fifth in this postscript. <u>Food</u> will be that fifth <u>F</u> word. <u>Friends, Fun, Forward, Focused,</u> and some really great <u>Food</u> sounds like a party of <u>Friends</u> having Fun in a <u>Forward Focused</u> way to me! Put it together and you'll have all the ingredients and the perfect environment in which you can move to action in the direction of your own self-care.

CHAPTER
13

READY, SET, GO!

*"I love that every day I get to decide where I'm going
and what I'm going to do when I get there.
I am my own experiment. I am my own work of art."*
Lorrie Forde

Everyone in your community of support is on this journey together. You all share the goal of healthy self-care and you all like the idea that it will be **Fun**. Take turns facilitating the group and leading the conversation. Take turns hosting the gatherings. Getting together (whether in person or via technology) is intended to support your self-care—not hinder it by adding stress and just one more thing to do, so share the responsibility. Create the vibe you want. You might choose to have everyone bring something for a potluck. Delegating roles can lighten the load, and rotating locations could add to the **Fun**. Whatever you choose to do, be sure to use the assignments and activities in this book as your **Foundation**. That will make it easy for you to stay intentional and moving **Forward** toward your common goal of self-care. Build on the **Foundation** that this book provides in ways that serve your own unique group. Adjust activities to fit the interests and resources of your group. Draw on one another's network of connections—there might be a great guest you could invite to one of your gatherings. Listen closely and pay attention to the quieter members of the group—they may have a great idea for your next get-together.

In the famous words of the popular athletic brand Nike, all that's left to do now is, "Just do it!"

Group Activity #1

> Group Activities are designed to encourage interactivity. Choose one person to act as the Facilitator. They will keep things moving _Forward_ and _Focused_ on the activity's outcome. Plan to _Focus_ on just one of the Group Activities at each gathering.

Setting the stage for your group's success is critical. Each group is different and will come up with its own set of unique group norms (rules). There are a few norms that are non-negotiable so I've started the list with those. Spend your first gathering coming up with the rest and making sure there is a shared commitment to confidentiality and support. The number of spaces below does not dictate how many group norms you will come up with. These are the rules that your group will agree upon and that will act as your guideposts as you move **Forward**. You may have only one or two beyond the four that I've suggested or your list may extend well beyond the twelve lines on this page. You may even discover that you will need to come back and revisit this exercise at a later date when something you hadn't considered presents itself. Perhaps this will also be a good time to talk about logistics such as how often you will meet. Even frequency of meetings deserves to be discussed as each group member will have unique demands on their time. Creating opportunity for everyone to have a voice will help satisfy the group norms of respect for each other and a willingness to listen.

What is said in the gathering stays in the gathering (confidentiality). _____

The environment will be respectful. _____

Each person will be willing to share. _____

Each person will be willing to listen. _____

_____

_____

_____

_____

_____

_____

_____

Group Activity #2

Now that the stage is set it's time to bring the cookie jar analogy to life. This is where that analogy will really begin to make sense. This activity is all about the jar (you). **Take your time with this activity**. Understanding where you are today with your level of self-care is going to serve you well as you consider where you want be on that self-care scale. And of course, making sure there is plenty of time on the agenda for **Fun** is also a priority!

Choose one person to lead the group in this visualization exercise. (*Note to visualization leader: go slowly with the questions. Allow your group plenty of time to "see" the image and find their own answers to the questions you are asking. Your job here is to hold the space with some silence for your group. The silence seems longer to you than it does to them.*)

Close your eyes, visualize your cookie jar, and consider these questions.

- What does it look like?
- How big is it?
- How **Full** is it?
- Is it empty?
- If there are any cookies in it—what kind are they?
- How many different types of cookies are there in your jar?
- What might be the advantages or disadvantages of having more than one type of cookie in your jar?
- When do you refill your cookie jar?

- Do you wait till it's empty with nothing other than a few crumbs in the bottom or do you top it up often?
- Do your cookies ever get stale?
- What do you think about that?

Open your eyes and discuss your answers in groups of five or fewer. Consider how you **Felt** during the visualization, what you're thinking and **Feeling** now that you're sharing your cookie-jar answers with others, and whether this exercise was easy or difficult and why. Ask others in the group how they might respond differently to this activity if they were to do it over again. Would their answers be the same if they did it again in just a few minutes, a month from now, or even next year? Consider how their answers impact you. Consider your own answers to these same questions. What are some of the factors that might cause someone to change their answers to the cookie jar questions? Remember to **take your time**—your insight and honesty at this stage will help you get really clear on what your **Favourite** cookies (self-care strategies) are.

Personal Assignment #1

Personal Assignments are something you will want to do on your own, in private, at times when you won't be interrupted and in a place where you Feel relaxed and comfortable. Personal Assignments will help prepare you for the conversations that will be on the agenda the next time your group meets.

Carve out a minimum of thirty minutes and create a quiet space for yourself. Bring this book as well as paper and pen. Write down a minimum of ten cookies (self-care strategies), things you currently do or would like to do for your own self-care. If you can come up with more than ten—do so—keep going till you run out of ideas. Some of you will find this exercise easier than others will. I once had a client who was not able to write down even three at her first try. Over time and with support she was able to come up with many more ideas and now she puts them into action as she practises healthy self-care on a daily basis.

Group Activity #3

> *As noted above, this is a time that the work you completed for Personal Assignment #1 will inform your readiness to participate in this Group Activity.*

- In groups of five or fewer, discuss what **Feeds** you, what kind of cookies (self-care strategies) you want in your jar.
- Make sure everyone has a list of cookies they can **Feel** good about. Use the energy of your group to come up with even more ideas.
- Talk about which ones would be your top three strategies if you were asked to prioritize them, and explain how and why you came to that decision.
- If there are more than five people in your group, mix up the two groups and repeat the discussion/exercise.

Group Activity #4

Dos and Don'ts for this activity:

- Do listen carefully. Listen with more than your ears—use your eyes, your intuition, and your heart to hear your partner's truth. Your goal here is to be a contributing thinking partner. I like to think of it as three levels of listening.
  - » On the surface, we're just listening for ourselves, listening for things that are of interest to us.

» Go a little deeper into the listening pool and we begin to listen for both of us. At this level, we are paying attention to points that will serve both our interests.
» When we dive all the way down we get to that deepest level of listening and, at this point, we are **Focused** on listening for the other person. We've moved from listening for me to listening for us and finally to listening for you.

- Do allow for silence—silence really can be golden when you're listening to someone.
- Do ask open questions. Questions that begin with *how* or *what* are good choices.
- Don't ever interrupt until your partner has had time to see their own barriers. Listening all the way through is the best gift we can give to our partner.
- Don't judge.

Now that the rules are clearly understood it's time to move into the action. Keep these dos and don'ts in mind as you move through all of the activities in this book. In addition to this book, strengthening your skill as a listener will serve you well in all aspects of your life. Whether you're listening to a **Friend**, your child, or a colleague at work, effective listening is a powerful tool.

- Break into groups of two or three.
- Share your list of cookies with your partner(s) and tell them honestly, what's stopping you from baking those cookies.
- Look at each self-care strategy individually and consider it with the attention and time it deserves.
- Now let your partner do the same.
- Remember the risks of should-ing (being obliged to do something) and the three-finger rule (if you're should-ing on another, there are three fingers pointing back at you).
- Depending on how many people are in your group, swap partners and go through the exercise again.
- Get really clear on what the true barriers are so you'll be better able to jump those hurdles when the time comes.
- Return to the larger group and share your personal ahas as you choose.

Personal Assignment #2

- Create a quiet space and time for yourself when you'll have a minimum of thirty minutes to review and reflect on those last two group activities.
- Prioritize your top three self-care strategies (cookies).
- Be clear about why you chose them as your top three.

Group Activity #5

- In groups of two or three, discuss what you need to support you to **Follow** through and bake your top three cookies.
- Consider the barriers you identified in the last activity.
- Tell your partner(s) where you rank yourself on a scale from one to ten in terms of your level of commitment to baking those top three cookies.
- If either of you rank yourself at less than a ten, discuss what it would take for you to get to a place where you could rank yourself at ten.
- Come back to the larger group and share your learning from this activity as you choose.

Personal Assignment #3

Now that you've had some practice, finding that thirty minutes for private time should be getting a little easier so work toward taking sixty minutes this time as you work through these seven steps.

1. Bring a paper and pen (and don't forget this book) so you can write down your contract with yourself.
2. Consider all the work that you've done in terms of getting clear on what your current self-care practices include.
3. Celebrate your progress!

Don't skip this important step—how will you celebrate? Being intentional in our plan to celebrate milestones along the way are as important as setting a goal was in the beginning. Some of my celebratory strategies include

* *a walk on a sunny day,*
* *dedicated time for a movie or a good book,*
* *gold stars on a calendar,*
* *lunch out with a friend, and*
* *a fancy coffee.*

4. Review the priorities you set for self-care practices as you move **Forward** from here.
5. Reflect on the potential barriers and the strategies you've identified to overcome them.
6. Ask yourself these questions:

When will I commit to "baking" and how will I hold myself accountable?

_____

_____

_____

_____

Where will I find the motivation to maintain my stick-with-it-ness when times get tough and barriers pop up?

_____

_____

_____

_____

_____

7.   While it's **Fresh** in your mind—use that pen and paper to write out the entire contract or fill in the blanks on the next page. Be specific with your commitments and limit yourself to a maximum of three. **Focus** on setting yourself up for success.

By _____ (date) I will have done _____ (#) things that "**Feed**" me. They are

_____

_____

_____

_____

_____

I will hold myself accountable to **Following** through on this plan with these actions:

_____

_____

_____

_____

_____

Signed: _____

Dated: _____

Group Activity #6

- Share your signed contract with the rest of your community of support.
- Talk about how easy it is to see when someone else's jar is running low and how you'll transfer that ability as you check in on your own jar regularly.
- Discuss the statement: "We can't make more time; we can only TAKE it, so plan the plan, **Follow** the plan, and let the results take care of themselves."
- Celebrate your success and the success of your **Friends**.

CHAPTER

14

THE LAW OF ACTION

"It takes as much energy to wish as it does to plan."
Eleanor Roosevelt

It is my belief that when intention meets potential and action is added into the mix there is every reason to believe that we will achieve the life we want.

I suspect you've all heard about the Law of Attraction (LOA) and if you haven't, pull out your laptop or smartphone as Mr. Google has an abundance of information and other resources to share. I've attended LOA workshops and even read more than one book on the subject. Law of Attraction gurus encourage us to visualize what we want and then to go beyond that visualization to a place of imagining what it would **Feel** like to have present in our lives that which we've visualized. They suggest that we create vision boards that consist of a collage of images or words that describe our vision and then to strategically place that board in a location where we'll see it several times each day. The belief is that each time we catch sight of the images on the board our subconscious will go to work manifesting the reality in which what we desire shows up for us.

As you enter into the process of connecting with your goal, the closer you can get to **Feeling** as though your goal is something you're meant to do or be and that you've already achieved it, the closer you are to seeing that goal actualized. Couple that with the fact that when we're living authentically we are virtually unstoppable and you have a powerful recipe for Goal Getting. Thinking in terms of "Goal Getting" versus "Goal Setting" also helps to propel us in the direction we want to go. Goal Getting is where the goal setter shifts from the vision to the action that will result in achieving the goal they're **Focused** on.

In my **Family** of origin, visualization was a regular practice from the time I was a very small child. My earliest memories of invoking the Law of Attraction are from when I was about four years old. My sister, who was two at the time, and I would often go with our dad as he ran errands in the car. Without exception, as soon as we got into the vehicle, our **Father** would say, "Get to work, girls" and we knew exactly what we were supposed to do. It was our job (and we took it very seriously) to visualize a parking spot at the **Front** of whatever store we were en route to. Interestingly, it worked and as you might imagine, our young minds took all of the credit for the vacant parking stall. As an adult, I cannot thank my **Father** enough for creating this deep-rooted belief in the power of the mind and as my **Friends** and **Family** will attest—the parking spots continue to manifest.

While I still subscribe to the concept and practice of visualization, I also believe that it is just the **First** step in achieving goals and that being able to link visualization to action is the real key for success. This is where Newton's Laws of Motion, and specifically the Law of Action (and reaction) resonate for me.

Picture that row of five steel balls hanging in a frame—it's actually called "Newton's cradle." Picking up two balls at one end and letting them swing **Forward** to collide with the adjacent balls causes the two balls at the far end of the row to be propelled out only to return and repeat the action in reverse order again and again until eventually the momentum dies down and the balls lie quietly once again. If there were seven balls in the cradle and you picked up two from one end and dropped them, the two on the opposite end would spring to action. If you only swung one ball then just one ball at the other end of the series would move.

For me, this law of equal and opposite action and reaction is the next step in the visualization process. Visualization is one critical stage; the ability to move into imagining how it would **Feel** to already have the outcome is another; and the total unlimited commitment to moving to action is the third. When that **First** ball is dropped, its commitment goes a hundred percent to **Following** through, and the subsequent result is guaranteed—the ball on the other end will respond accordingly. It is our own willingness to enter a state of unlimited commitment and willingness to jump to conscious action in the moment of opportunity that is where the Law of Action meets intentional Goal Setting: Goal Getting. For me the Law of Action is paramount in achieving goals and making dreams a reality.

Conscious action is just that—a pre-planned choice to seize opportunities as they present themselves, to deliberately say yes while the window of opportunity is open, and to maintain the momentum by continuing to be intentional and aware of the action you can take that will keep you moving **Forward** along the path to your goals and dreams.

One task at a time is all you need to tackle. Just like you talked about in Group Activity #6—Plan the plan, **Follow** the plan, and let the results take care of themselves. Detaching from the outcome is important. Hold on to your passion, move to action, and get out of the way till the next step is presented to you. Signs you're on the right path are that you **Feel** in sync with the universe and that things seemingly find their way to you with little or no effort on your part. Connecting with your true authentic self is a key ingredient in the recipe for creating enough space for everything you desire to find its way to you.

Letting go of the outcome and staying in the present can be challenging as we are a culture that likes to be in control. Help yourself and the rest of your group to stay on track by **Focusing** on just one step at a time. Think in terms of the image below.

Objective ⇨ Intention ⇨ Action ⇨ Success.

This step-by-step picture of Goal Getting does even more than just help us to stay **Focused**. It also assists in making the decision to move **Forward** in the **First** place. Looking at anything in its entirety can be overwhelming so breaking it down to bite-sized pieces just makes sense. The old question of "How do you eat an elephant?" with the answer "One bite at a time." is based on exactly the same principle. If we look at the whole elephant, there is no way that we will ever believe we could eat the whole thing. However, once we look at that elephant as nothing more than the sum of several manageable meals, the task becomes just that much more doable.

> *Warning—even though I cited Food as a really good F word, this reference to eating elephants is not intended to encourage readers to actually eat elephants!*

This same concept is used with great success by many as they aim for and intentionally work toward achieving their targets and goals. Those engaged in weight-loss strategies stay on track by **Focusing** on weekly objectives versus the overall goal. People dealing with addiction think in terms of making it through the week or if that's too long, they **Focus** on making it through the day and if that's still too long, they break that day into hours and those hours into minutes and those minutes into seconds. Those seconds and minutes turn into hours, days, weeks, months, and eventually years of success.

It's really just that simple. Simple is not always easy. Break the goal down into bite-sized pieces, visualize your success, enjoy imagining how it will **Feel** to have achieved that success, and move to action one step at a time.

See it. **Feel** it. Do it!

It is always important to celebrate your successes along the way too. As you achieve milestones along the path toward your overall goal, you might choose to revisit a strategy that was and still is effective with kids.

Aren't we really all just kids at heart when it comes right down to it?

A sticker system works well for me and many others I know. We identify the key milestones in writing, and as we pass them, we give ourselves a sticker to honour the accomplishment. I keep my sticker chart on the **Front** of my fridge and find that its visibility really motivates me to stay on track and move **Forward** in the direction of my overall goal. The stickers I give myself along the way are proof that I'm making progress.

"You can live your life out of circumstance or you can live it out of vision."
Unknown

Group Activity #7

- Regardless of whether you're meeting face to face or via technology—wherever they are, everyone will need a blank piece of letter-sized paper (8.5" x 11") and a pen or pencil.
- Ask each person to mark small X's anywhere on the paper that they choose to. Each X on the paper represents a significant goal they see as having accomplished in their life.
- Tell each person to be sure to include all those important milestones. (Examples might be

completing school, a healthy relationship, having kids, surviving a particularly challenging day/event, etc.)

- Now look at how much blank space there is on the paper compared to the little X's that represent each of those life achievements and goals.
- Ask each person to consider that the space between the X's is their life journey and consider how much more white space there is in contrast to the space the X's take up on the page.

Discuss as a group

- The value of having a goal to work toward.
- The risk(s) of becoming too attached to outcomes.
- The value of staying present in the moment and **Focusing** on the process.

When I did this activity myself and considered how much white space there was left on my paper, it made me think what a good representation the blank space is of how much more time I spend on getting to a goal than the actual moment when I achieve that goal. From that realization, it was just a short step to the awareness of how much value there is in staying present in the moment, rather than worrying about what may or may not ever materialize. It was a great reminder to trust that if I Follow the action plan I've developed for achieving a specific goal, I will achieve it, regardless of how much time I spend thinking or worrying about it.

CHAPTER
15

CORE CONNECTION

Each of us is the architect of our own unique life. We have the right and the responsibility to design our lives in order that they look just like we want them to look. So, if your life looks like anything less than you'd imagined—change it!

This is easier said than done though.

Connecting to our core purpose, our heart's desire, our passion is simultaneously simple and incredibly challenging. Simple because it requires nothing more than truth and desire, and challenging because it requires honesty and action.

Each of us has hopes and desires. Uncovering the inspiration to connect with our core purpose can be elusive. Be kind to yourself—you deserve to get what you want. It's when we align desire with opportunity and intention that we are best able to move to action in the direction of our goal.

We know that "like attracts like" and we can wrap our heads around the concept of "be what you want and you'll get what you are." In addition, the reality is that everything around us is changing all the time.

> *Think about how time-lapse photography is able to capture the magic of change.*

We too are changing; embrace that truth and create change that works for you. You have the power to make any dream come true. Be clear, be consistent, be committed, and move to action to create the reality you want. The answer to the questions of how to connect with your core is basically "Don't find your passion—live your passion!"

"Our bodies are our gardens to which our wills are gardeners."
William Shakespeare

Uncovering one's passion is a popular coaching topic among the clients I work with. It's easy for me to empathize with my clients on this topic as I too have spent considerable time on the question of what it is that I'm passionate about engaging in during my "me time." Some people seem to have such a clear picture of what they love to do. For some it's golf or sailing, others **Feel** a deep connection with exercising in the gym or running, and many are able to lose themselves in the making of music or other art forms. The common denominator these people all share is that they're passionate about whatever it is that they've chosen to do and for those of us who haven't yet been able to figure out just what our **Favourite** activities are—we continue to drool over the thought of someday getting to that place of knowing.

There have been times when I've thought about the possibility that I may be trying too hard or overthinking the question about what I want to do with my **Free** time. Perhaps my definition of "passion" is too idealistic. Possibly, I want to be head-over-heels passionate about everything. I know I enjoy engaging in a host of **Fun** activities and I think it's **Fair** to say that I'm passionate about travel in particular. Travel stimulates me on every level. I get immense pleasure from the overall experience in spite of the challenges that often go hand in hand with travel to distant lands. I learn about new cultures, see new sights, meet new **Friends**, taste delicious new **Foods**, attempt unfamiliar languages, come away with a host of powerful memories, and, in hindsight, see that my worldview has been enhanced and deepened.

How realistic is it to think that I can engage in that kind of travel as often as I'd like to, in order to do something I'm passionate about? Realistically, those trips are at best once per year. What about the other eleven months?

I've created a reality where I enjoy working in a field that I'm passionate about. I am also incredibly grateful that occasionally I'm able to incorporate my passion for travel into my work as a coach through both client retreats and technology that allows me to meet with clients regardless of where they are in the world.

The **Fact** that I've found work that is very meaningful for me and that truly connects me with my core purpose leaves me curious about why my **Free** time is such a challenge. And if that isn't the epitome of a first-world problem, I don't know what is! But I live in the first world and so my **Free** time activities find their way into the **Focus** of some of my intentional planning and goal setting. Through this intentional action, I continue to deepen my understanding of just what my learning on this front might be.

Could it be that enjoyment of a **Fun** activity is as good as it gets? Am I settling if it's anything less than the all-encompassing engagement I **Feel** while travelling to distant lands? Or is passion nothing more than enjoyment coupled with **Focus**? When I'm travelling in unfamiliar territory, it's a **Fact** that all of my attention is spent **Focused** on the experience. I am a hundred percent living in the moment. Perhaps that requirement to be alert, **Focused**, and completely engaged in the present is where the passion is born—an interesting concept that I will continue to explore as I seek out activities that I can do throughout the year and that stimulate me in the same way that travel does.

Or is "passion" even the right word to use when I'm searching for something to do? Perhaps it would be better if I were to reframe "passion" to "purpose" or even "interest" and use my curious nature to open the door to new perspectives about passion. What if instead of searching for my passion I simply engaged in activities I enjoy and then got passionate about doing them? Would the result not be the same? I'm pretty sure that I'd still be **Feeling** the passion regardless of whether the passion or the interest came first.

> *Perhaps connecting with my core purpose is not so much what I do as how I do it. More Food for thought....*

What activities do you most look **Forward** to?

_____

_____

_____

_____

_____

Does anything about them leave you wanting more? If so, what?

_____

_____

_____

_____

How do those activities tie in with your core purpose and living your authentic life?

_____

_____

_____

_____

Where do core purpose, authentic life, and passion overlap?

_____

_____

_____

_____

What will you do today to deepen your understanding of what leaves you **Feeling** connected to your core purpose?

_____

_____

_____

_____

How can you leverage your skills and abilities to initiate action toward the milestones that mark the path to your heart's desire?

_____

_____

_____

_____

_____

How will you use your unique personality to your advantage on this journey?

_____

_____

_____

_____

How have you made this **Focused** Q & A activity **Fun** for yourself?

_____

_____

_____

_____

_____

What role will your network (your **Friends**) play in this process?

_____

_____

_____

_____

_____

CHAPTER

16

BEGIN BEFORE YOU'RE READY

Having a clearly defined goal is both a smart thing to have and a powerful place to begin. In a perfect world we would all know exactly where we're headed at all times and if I'm to be completely truthful, there have been times when I've not been a hundred percent clear on what I want as my ultimate goal and certainly not clear on how I'm going to get there. While it may be true that if you don't have a clear plan to **Follow**, you might end up somewhere other than where you want to be, it's also true that waiting till everything is in perfect order could be leaving it a little too long.

My intention with this chapter is to invite you to keep it simple and to just get moving. Adjustments can be made along the way, and in **Fact**, by waiting until we're actually face to face with a challenge, our ability to successfully name and overcome the barrier is that much greater. Who knows—some of those barriers we imagine may never even materialize.

How do we begin when we don't know where to begin? The answer to this is simple and again—not necessarily easy. Begin by doing anything! Moving to action will invoke Newton's three Laws of Motion and before you know it, you'll be on your way. Newton may not entirely agree with the overly simplistic way I interpret his laws here, but for the purposes of this context, I'll walk my talk, move to action with my definition, and beg **Forgiveness** later. The **First** law basically states that nothing will change until something changes. The second references the importance of size. For example, the bigger the hurdle— the more force required to clear the barrier. The third and final law in this series of stages involved in affecting change simply says that when we move to action there will be a consequence.

Simply invoking Newton's laws won't get you to exactly where you want to go. It will, however, begin the process and provide you with information and stimulation that will help you plan your next step. While all three of Newton's laws are vitally important steps in the process of getting to your goal, it will be the third law that helps keep you moving after you've started. It's hard to stop something that's already in motion. In **Fact**, it's easier to move with the momentum of the action than it is to resist it.

There are eight steps to starting:

1. interest in moving **Forward**,
2. intention to **Follow** through,
3. desire for a goal-**Focused** outcome,
4. courage to **Face** the barriers as they come up,
5. willingness to stay in the moment,
6. energy to keep moving **Forward**,
7. a positive attitude, and
8. party-planning skills so you can commit to celebrating your milestones and your success in style at the same time as you move to action.

So, shift out of neutral and start now!

"Be a beginner at something."
Steve Jobs

CHAPTER
17

COMMAND AND CONTROL

The **Focus** for this chapter presented itself to me during the summer as I worked on writing this book while doing double duty as grandma to two very active and creative boys. It's a rare treat that I have both grandsons together and as there is a five-year age difference between them, it's not often that they find ways they can play together. This day was perfect though—we were at the beach and the boys had recruited a group of like-minded fellows. "Army" was the game of the day, and it was in that context that I overheard one boy say, "Go to command and control for your assignment as soon as you wake up."

The synchronicity of that part of their play with the content I was working on was interesting, to say the least, so I took it as a sign and wrote it down as something to consider for a chapter topic. This group of boys (ranging in age from five to ten years old) had the strategy to daily success all figured out. They simply had to get their orders at the start of the day and they'd be good to go. I had already incorporated the practice of "command and control" into my life and yet I'd never had a name for it.

This practice of checking in each morning to be intentional about the day ahead is a popular strategy that has worked for many. For me, it's been an effective tool for ensuring daily self-care practices don't slip through the cracks of my busy life.

I'd heard it referred to as a "power hour" or "daily planning" and neither of those had really resonated for me the way this command-and-control analogy did. I could actually picture myself as the commander issuing directives that were based on logic and goals. The name didn't invite emotional attachment to the activities and even that **Fact** was in support of **Following** through to get it done. No drama—just intention, action, and accomplishment.

Simply put "command and control" is a definite block of time dedicated to a specific set of functions each and every day. This committed time is non-negotiable and takes priority over all else. It is a commitment to self-care and in no way is it selfish. I work to make it **Fun** and sometimes I bring my **Friends** into it by sharing my ahas with them. My command-and-control time is very **Focused** and when people ask me how I manage to maintain my healthy self-care, I'm able to respond with the truth, that I get it done in tiny bite-sized pieces.

Some choose to dedicate an hour (or more) each morning. My command-and-control time has evolved to be a perfect match for my life at a maximum of thirty minutes every weekday. There are times when I think about growing that thirty minutes to a **Full** hour but for me at this stage in my life, thirty minutes is perfect!

Here's how I spend my dedicated command-and-control time each day:

- fifteen minutes meditating or thinking mindfully,
- five minutes planning for my health and **Fitness** goals for the day,
- five minutes planning my **Free** time goal for the day, and
- five minutes for intentional reflection and gratitude.

Yes, I dedicate time for health, **Fitness**, and **Free** time every day. I use part of my command-and-control time to plan how I want to use that dedicated time. As part of my self-care practice, I remind myself that I am the one making all the decisions for command and control—I am the commander and completely in control. I give myself permission to choose to be **Flexible** with my dedicated daily time(s) when that **Feels** like the right thing to do. I might decide to make activities longer or shorter than originally planned. For example, if my health and **Fitness** goal for the day was to spend a total of twenty minutes on an activity, I could either go for a twenty-minute walk or I could do one minute on the stairs five times throughout the day plus ten minutes on the bike as well as a short walk to the mailbox. In the end, I would still have completed my goal of twenty minutes and I would have stayed true to my personal preference for flexibility and variety. Alternately, I might merge activities and targets with one another or I might get really creative with my definition of what **Free** time looks like or what can fall under the heading of health and **Fitness**. One example of merging my goals that I often enjoy is to listen to music (a **Free**-time activity) while I engage in my **Fitness** commitment. And on some days my **Free** time takes the form of a walk so on those days I'm meeting my **Fitness** target at the same time as I'm attaining my **Free** time goal.

I set myself up for success by making my daily goals doable. For example, I put my exercise bike right in the middle of my living room so I cannot avoid seeing it every time I walk by. I also plan to spend several short periods of time (three to five minutes) on the bike so it's never long enough to get boring. One of the things I discovered in the self-awareness portion of my self-care journey is that I love variety and spontaneity. I've also learned that without having committed time it's too easy not to **Follow** through and to have my self-care practice slip lower on my priority list. Life is busy and as commander I have the responsibility to do my best to plan for every possible scenario. Busyness is no excuse and cannot take priority over me and my self-care plan. To ensure that doesn't happen I've had to find a way to combine variety, spontaneity, and planning. The short list above that describes how I spend my command-and-control time is what my daily action planning process looks like.

Now it's your turn. Reflect back on some of the new insights and self-awarenesses you've gained as you've worked your way through the assignments and activities in this book. At the same time, draw on the self-awareness you've earned through your lifetime of experience. No matter how long your life—it's your lifetime. Be proud of all that you've earned and learned already. Use that awareness to guide your responses to the questions below. You know better than anyone what your preferences and needs are. Use that knowledge to customize your command-and-control time into something that is a perfect fit for you.

How might I spend my command-and-control time?

_____

_____

_____

_____

What are the potential benefits of dedicating time for this type of intentional planning?

_____

_____

_____

_____

How long would I like to spend each day strategizing for self-care?

_____

_____

_____

_____

_____

How much time will I dedicate to putting that self-care plan into practice each day?

_____

_____

_____

_____

What are some of the spin-off benefits that might materialize through this command-and-control strategy?

_____

_____

_____

_____

What might get in the way of me **Following** through with my plan?

_____

_____

_____

_____

What can I do to mitigate those potential barriers?

_____

_____

_____

_____

When will I begin this practice?

_____

_____

_____

_____

How will I hold myself accountable for **Following** through?

_____

_____

_____

Who might I enlist to help me stick with my plan?

_____

_____

_____

What milestones will I set and how will I celebrate my success as I reach them?

_____

_____

_____

"I am right where I am as a direct result of the choices I make."
Lynda Green

CHAPTER
18

YOUR LIFE IS YOUR JOB

Do you agree with the statement in this title that your life is your job? When I **First** considered this as a chapter title, I spent some time thinking about it. As a baby boomer, my strong work ethic helps define me. As a **Family** member or **Friend**, my strong work ethic (*aka* commitment to others) is an important part of who I am in a relationship. As a coach, my strong work ethic drives my high standards as I work for my clients and it is part of the reason my business is successful. So when I thought about my life being my job—it gave me a new context in which to think about my responsibility to myself. In **Fact**, if my life is my job and if I truly am my own boss then I am also my own employer and my life is my business. As I consider the responsibility I take when running a company, I realize that I am extremely intentional about ensuring my business success. Practices such as Risk Management reviews and both short- and long-term Strategic Planning ensure the health of my organization. So how is it that I'm not always as intentional in my role as Chief Executive Officer in my life?

I know with all certainty that I am great in my roles of employee, employer, **Family** member,

Friend, and colleague. And if I'm completely honest, I think there are times when I may not score as high on the self-care scale as I do on my external work ethic practices. That's not to say that I don't know how to take care of myself; it's more about our culture, my upbringing, the generation I was born into, and my willingness to do whatever needs to be done. I can think of many times over the years when the doing of a particular thing came at the expense of my self-care, and in hindsight, I have to say that in those moments I wasn't doing a very good job of looking after my life. I also know that I made those choices for reasons, some of which were out of my control.

I'm not going to beat myself up about any of that. It is in the past and I am really only interested in going **Forward**. However, I will carry the awareness I gained through those past experiences **Forward** with me and use the learning from them the next time I'm faced with having to choose where my self-care and I sit on my priority list.

Perhaps I will find a way to fit some **Fun** into the job at hand, or maybe I'll look for a way to include some **Friends** in the process. Most certainly though I will be aware of the need to **Focus** on the question of whether or not I am doing as well on my own self-care ranking as I am on the traditional performance appraisal from the workplace or **Feedback** from **Family** and **Friends**.

Whether you work inside or outside the home, we all know that our culture values a strong work ethic. Some of you will be self-employed, others will be leaders within an organization, and a few of you will be in transition while looking for work. Whatever your circumstance, respond to the questions from your unique perspective.

What are some of the qualities you describe as providing evidence of a good employee? (If you're self-employed, a homemaker, or engaged in a job search describe your expectations of yourself.)

_____

_____

_____

_____

What would an employer say about your work ethic? (Regardless of whether you're self-employed, in a workplace, or are currently between jobs—you can imagine what an employer would say about you.)

_____

_____

_____

_____

How would that same employer rate your level of self-care? (If you don't have an employer at the moment, consider how your colleagues, **Friends**, and **Family** would rate your level of self-care. If you're the employer, how would your employees rate you?)

_____

_____

_____

_____

And now for the big question. If your life is your job then how committed are you to moving in the direction of creating a reality where your self-care ranking is at least as high as your workplace score? Or to put it another way—would you want to work for you?

_____

_____

_____

_____

What changes might you make to become a better "employer"?

_____

_____

_____

_____

CHAPTER
19

WHERE ARE YOU ON YOUR PRIORITY LIST?

These last few questions about work ethic and qualities we look for in a workplace lead us straight to this very powerful one: "Where are you on your priority list?" This is one of those potentially emotional topics that often come up when I'm working with clients who are experiencing some frustration with their ability to achieve their goal(s). Typically, those same clients are surprised to discover that they're either very low on their priority list and—in more than a few cases—not even showing up on it at all!

Where are you on your priority list? Are you like so many others who say they're not even on it? Do tears spring to your eyes or does your throat tighten as you read this question? Does a vision of your empty cookie jar flash before your eyes? If so, know that this awareness and these tears represent the truth and they let you know that you've just uncovered an opportunity to move **Forward** in the direction of your choice.

Considering where we rank on our priority list is a great exercise—not because the answer needs to be dissected under a microscope—because it brings **Fantastic** awareness to a gap that may exist. If we're not high enough on our own list, how can we possibly expect to be able to achieve any of the goals we set for ourselves when one of our goals is self-care? The irony becomes almost laughable!

In coaching, we **Focus Forward** at all times so in the case of someone who discovers they're not very high on their own priority list we would look at how that new awareness fits for them. If they say it does fit, then so be it. If they say it doesn't, then we **Focus** on how to move **Forward** through a series of coaching questions that build on one another. This new awareness repeatedly brings commitment to move to action and initiate new choices in support of a specific desired outcome.

Over time and with practice, I've learned that by being intentional with my self-care I can create a reality where I'm showing up on my priority list all the time.

On a scale of 1 to 10 where 1 is "I'm number one on my list" and 10 is "I'm last on the list," where are you on your priority list? Circle your answer.

1   2   3   4   5   6   7   8   9   10

How do you **Feel** about the ranking you just gave yourself?

_____

_____

_____

_____

_____

> *If you'd like to see any change to your status on that priority list, please continue and we'll have a mini coaching session. There is no rush so take your time. Don't think about your answers too long though. Likely, your initial response will be the truth and you deserve the truth. As well, the best thing about a mind is that it can change so if you decide you want to change one of your responses at any time—you can.*

Where would you like to be on your priority list?

_____

_____

_____

_____

How realistic or doable is that?

_____

_____

_____

_____

What needs to happen for you to move up higher on that list?

_____

_____

_____

_____

What do you need to do to make that happen?

_____

_____

_____

_____

What might get in the way of your doing that?

_____

_____

_____

_____

What could you do to minimize those barriers?

_____

_____

_____

_____

On a scale of 1 to 10 where 1 is "not at all" and 10 is "very committed," circle how committed you are to **Following** through with doing whatever it takes to move yourself higher on your priority list.

1   2   3   4   5   6   7   8   9   10

When are you prepared to move to action on these things you've just described?

_____

_____

_____

_____

How will you hold yourself accountable to **Following** through?

_____

_____

_____

_____

As is the case with all of the activities in this book, your willingness, honesty, and the time you're committing will provide you with a **Framework** you can work from. This **Framework** is a place for you to gain perspective and a clearer view of your goal(s) as you begin to shift to a place that is closer to where you'd like to be as you move **Forward**.

CHAPTER

20

YOU CAN'T MAKE TIME, BUT YOU CAN TAKE IT!

Think of how often you've said, "I'm going to have to make time for that," or "I'm so sorry, I just couldn't make the time." Whenever I hear anyone say anything about "making" time, I call "B.S."! We all know there are only twenty-four hours in a day and none of us can "make" any more.

What was your reaction to my calling "B.S."? I fear that it may have been offensive to some and if so, I apologize. My intent was not to offend; it was rather to really drive home the <u>Fact</u> that it's all up to you—your choice. If we were working together in person, I'd be able to couch the "B.S." comment by prefacing it with something like, "with due respect," or "no offence intended." Here, though, we are at a distance and as we move through this process of strategizing for self-care, I am working toward leaving you in a space where you commit to take a hundred percent ownership of the responsibility for that task before we get to the end of this book.

While we can't "make" time, we can certainly "take" time. If something is high enough on our priority list to warrant us fitting it into our already busy schedules, then I encourage you to say it like it is and commit to taking the time to do whatever "it" is. If it is not important enough to earn your valuable time, simply say "no" at the outset and save yourself and everyone else some of the stress of unmet promises.

Time Management is another popular topic requested by my clients. I often think we could re-name it Self-Management though, as that might be a more accurate title.

When I'm working with a client who, by their own admission, is over-promising and under-delivering in their lives I have a pretty good hunch that it is easier for them to say "yes" than it is for them to say "no" to people—even when "no" is what they want to say. To support them in achieving their goal of changing that pattern, I have even been known to strike a little below the belt by having them recognize their desire to take care of others. I do this simply by asking them to put themselves in the other person's place and imagine how that person will **Feel** when the original "yes" turns into a "sorry" at the eleventh hour. This tactic along with a question or two about how logic and logistics also fit into the equation can work wonders in shedding some light on the downside of over-promising.

As a coach, I am constantly searching for ways to form questions for my clients that will encourage them to plant tiny seeds of thoughtful consideration for themselves—seeds that will germinate over time and eventually blossom into **Full-blown** plans of action once they're ready to move **Forward** in achieving their goal.

When a client tells me they're tired of overcommitting and they don't want to **Feel** as though they're unable to keep up with all that they have to do any longer—you know that "stop the world I want to get off" **Feeling**—it opens the door for me to ask them to describe exactly what they'd like their life to look like instead. I explain that the more specific they can be at this point the easier it will be for them to see the target they're aiming for as we move **Forward** toward their goal.

Coaching questions such as "When you say 'yes' to something, what are you saying 'no' to?" or "How would it **Feel** to under-promise and over-deliver instead?" really resonate for those clients working on managing their time. I appeal to their desire to take care of themselves and others by asking questions like, "You say that you're over-promising and under-delivering. How is that serving you? How is it serving the person to whom you are making the unmet promise?"

For those of you who fall into this category of choosing to say "yes" even when you'd rather say "no," I'm going to draw on a couple of images that I hope will speak to you. For both of them I'm going to ask you to imagine that you are a parent, even if you're not. The motivation for my request is that I want to tap into your emotional response as I believe that is where your desire to say "yes" is rooted.

The **First** image is one that takes place at the start of every airline flight. You and your toddler are buckled into your seats for a domestic flight. It's not a long trip and you foresee no challenges as your little one is sleeping peacefully. The flight attendant begins her routine instruction. She tells you where the doors are, that the floor lights will activate in case of emergency, that there is a floatation device under your seat, and—here it comes—the message that makes you cringe every time you hear it. Your logical mind tells you that it's true and yet you simply cannot imagine being able to do it—especially when it is your child who is sitting right beside you. Have you figured out what the instruction is yet? It's the one where the flight attendant says, "In the case of an emergency please put on your own oxygen mask **First** before helping anyone else around you." Logically, of course this is true. If you don't take care of yourself **First** there is no way you'll be of any help to the toddler sitting next to you. Still you resist the idea.

The next image is one that I saw on a television commercial. I have no memory of what the ad was for and, even so, the image will never leave me: it was so powerful. To make it more powerful, I will describe it as a visualization exercise. You and your child are on vacation and have rented a boat for the afternoon. You're on the water. You've made sure your child is safe. He is lathered in sunscreen and wearing the best life jacket money can buy. It's a gorgeous day and the sun is shining as you watch your child experience his **First** boating adventure. This is when the happy tranquil scene cuts to the next shot of your child alone in the boat safely ensconced in his life jacket while you are no longer in the picture—you've fallen overboard and your child is now orphaned and alone in a boat in the middle of nowhere!

The image is harsh and it pulls on my heartstrings. At the same time, it also drives home the importance of intentionally taking the time to take care of myself **First**. I know that doesn't mean I have to ignore or negate my responsibility and desire to care for others at the same time. It simply means that I have a responsibility to take as much care of myself as I'm providing to those around me.

So often, it really does boil down to the words we use. When I think of Time Management as self-management, I can see that the onus is on me to manage my time in a way that serves me and my responsibilities. When I consider under-promising and over-delivering, I think about the smiling faces versus the looks of disappointment that follow unfulfilled commitments. When I think about putting on my own life jacket (figuratively speaking), I know I'm putting myself high enough on the priority list to ensure I'm going to stay healthy, happy, and able to live a **Full** life, which includes **Fulfilling** my roles and responsibilities as a caregiver.

The question about what I'm saying "no" to when I'm saying "yes" to something else makes me wonder about whether there is a whole new world of **Fun** and **Friends** waiting for me once I stop trying to do the impossible—to "make" time.

"We must use time as a tool, not as a crutch."
John F. Kennedy

CHAPTER
21

FOLLOW THE LEADER

Think back to a time when as a child you **Felt** drawn to one **Friend** or a group of **Friends** whom you wanted to hang with—to be like. It's still that simple; take a look around you and **Find** those people who model the qualities you want to possess, the ones who live the life you aspire to, and those who leave you **Feeling** energized when you're in their presence.

Models come in all shapes and sizes so surround yourself with people who are living the life you want. Like-minded people support one another to reach for the stars. Alternatively, if you choose to spend time with people who settle for mediocrity, that's where you'll stay. It may be time to take a close look at which people in your life really support you and your intentional actions for self-care.

As I begin this chapter, I remember an assignment I had to complete for a course I was attending some time ago. I'll share that memory with you and encourage you to consider it for yourself as it was an interesting exercise that was much more impactful for me than I thought it might be at **First** glance. In a nutshell, I had to consider all of the people in my life and group them into four teams—A, B, C, and D. The A team would include those one or two people whom I trusted implicitly; the B team was larger and included the rest of those folks I considered to be solidly in my corner. The C team consisted of **Friends** and acquaintances, and the D team consisted of those people who weren't supporting me in my goals or in my life. Once I had all the teams assigned, I then had to deport my D team as it was no longer serving me—in **Fact**, it was draining me of critical life energy.

Some of you will choose to complete this whole exercise while others of you will just skim over the concept. Either way, my guess is that you'll quickly think of one or two people who are on your D team. What will you do with that new awareness? I often hear myself saying to my clients, "You can't un-know something, so what will you do now?"

Could it be that this is an opportunity for you to draw on your awareness about Newton's Laws of Motion? Perhaps deporting your D team will be easier than you think once the action is under way and the momentum is there to help carry it **Forward**. One consequence to the action of deportation is strengthening your team!

As I went through the stages of working with my editor, Nina, on this book, many of the _F_ words were challenged and my identification of "First" in "First glance" earlier in this chapter as a really good _F_ word caused a bit of dialogue. I wondered if this might be something you may question too and so I decided to give you a synopsis of how I came to the conclusion that it was in _Fact_ a really good _F_ word for me. Nina challenged that perhaps this _First_ wasn't all that good. I countered that had I stopped at _First_ glance, I never would have been drawn into the deeper learning of the exercise. I added that perhaps this is a bit like the question of whether a glass is half-full or half-empty, and that it is up to me how I choose to see it.

My choice was to view the _First_ glance as the _First_ step into an interesting and enlightening activity. For me, taking that _First_ step was critically important and it left me _Feeling_ good. Considering the way I describe my main method for determining good _F_ words at the beginning of this book; that was enough for me. Without that _First_ step, I would never have opened the door to this lesson. This _First_ glance was an example of me moving to action and invoking Newton's laws.

So dear reader—there you have it—a lot of work goes into the writing of a book and thanks to my amazing editor, some really good reflection too. Just as I got to decide that this "First" was a good _F_ word so do you get to decide which _F_ words work for you in your action plan for self-care.

Victoria's Story

This Friend gave me permission to share her story and I'm grateful for her generosity. She describes numerous moments that demonstrate so many of the topics we've covered in this book. Perhaps some of you will recognize yourself or someone you know in the words that follow.

Victoria's childhood was not terrible nor was it a bed of roses. She describes her life then and now as "pretty good." As a single mom of three pre-teens, she finds her work as a server in a restaurant demanding at times, but she doesn't dislike it.

Victoria is thirty-eight years old and lately her life seems to be flying by. For the **First** time ever she's been **Feeling** as though she might be settling for something less than she deserves. She always thought there would be lots of time to work toward her dreams. Now that forty is just around the corner, she can **Feel** some anxiety and fear of missing her chance if something doesn't happen soon.

What do you think about Victoria's current situation? Where do you think she's headed?

Another year would pass before Victoria would make the choice to change. Her change began with a stop at the local Visitor Information Centre where she met a volunteer named Tanya. Victoria **Felt** inspired by her conversation with Tanya. Not only did she receive the information she went into the Info Centre for, she also learned about some really great events coming up in the community over the next couple of months that sounded like they would be **Fun**. It had been a long time since Victoria had gone to anything **Fun** and now that she was thinking about it, she realized she had lost touch with many of her **Friends** too. Tanya had been so easy to talk to, so helpful, and so … **Friendly**. It had **Felt** so good and Victoria could **Feel** something shift inside.

The shift that Victoria **Felt** is where the hope was born (or reborn) for her that day. She began to believe that she could move beyond her "pretty good" life and toward something that looked more like what she'd dreamt of as a teen.

Victoria's dream had always been to be a veterinarian but—just as the shift she'd **Felt** was where hope had been reborn—this "but" is where fear and negative self-talk stepped in to hold her back.

> *"But" is one of those powerful words that I encourage my clients to reframe or work to eliminate from their vocabulary; it generally erases all that has come before it. In the case of Victoria, the thing her "but" worked to erase was her confidence and enthusiasm. Read on though—Victoria will find a way through this "but."*

This time of reborn hope **Felt** different, and Victoria was going to trust her intuition and dig deep into her desire to have some **Fun**. This would help her find the confidence to check out these local events she'd learned about at the Visitor Information Centre. She looked at the list of upcoming events and found three that were totally **Free** and that were also scheduled to take place on her days off.

Her two older kids didn't want to go to the **First** one, a farmers' market; however, the youngest one did and so the two of them set off. The sun was shining and it **Felt** good to be doing something different. Victoria couldn't figure out why she hadn't ever done this before now. There were a couple of street musicians she enjoyed listening to and the aromas wafting out of some of the stalls were making her mouth water.

Victoria was standing in a line to get some kind of crepe that looked amazing when she heard a voice say, "Hello."

It was Tanya, the **Friendly** woman from the Visitor Information Centre.

Victoria **Felt** herself smile in return and knew that something was different today. It was as though she was nineteen again and anything was possible.

The two women chatted as they enjoyed their crepes and watched Victoria's eight-year-old play with some **Friends** in the park right next to the market.

Victoria **Felt** intrigued by the **Fact** that she was again **Feeling** inspired by Tanya's positive attitude and infectious smile. It was as though Tanya had the world by the tail and Victoria wanted some of the same.

Before long, the conversation got around to the volunteer work Tanya was doing at the Visitor Centre. Tanya said there were oodles of opportunities to volunteer in the community and encouraged her new **Friend** to think about volunteering for something too. Tanya sounded excited as she said, "I love being able to help out and know that I'm making a difference." Victoria said she would think about it—and she did. In **Fact**, for some reason she couldn't get the idea out of her mind. So, on her next day off, she went back to the Visitor Centre to find out about volunteer opportunities. Tanya wasn't there this time. Instead, it was Greg, the volunteer for that day, and he was every bit as happy, helpful, and encouraging as Tanya had been.

Victoria took the list of volunteer opportunities home with her. It was long! She **Felt** inspired by her conversation with Greg. It was as though his and Tanya's positivity was contagious.

At dinner that night, Victoria told her kids about meeting Greg and bringing home a list of volunteer opportunities. The kids were far more interested than she thought they would be. They wanted to look at the list too, so she pulled it out and together they began to consider all the options.

You may already have guessed the wonderful outcome. It wasn't long before Victoria saw the opportunity for a volunteer worker at a local veterinary office. The veterinarian donates a block of time each week to caring for stray animals and they were in need of someone who could assist with the procedures during those times.

Victoria's eyes filled with tears as she **Felt** the flood of the memory of her childhood dream wash over her. She knew in her heart that her dream was about to become a reality.

Another year passed and Victoria had her fortieth birthday. She's still **Friends** with Tanya and she spends four hours each week volunteering in the animal hospital as a **Fully** trained veterinary assistant.

She often thinks of the day that she went to the Visitor Information Centre and met Tanya. Victoria knows that her life today is as happy and busy as she is. She's taking great care of herself as she gives herself the gift of time each week to live her passion working with animals. Who knows where it will lead. Meanwhile Victoria's life has moved from "pretty good" to "awesome!"

When she opened the door to doing something different, she invoked the Law of Attraction and, when she walked through it and took it to the next step, she became **Fully** engaged in the Law of Action. She saw what she wanted, she imagined what it would be like to do it, she moved to action, and she did it. This is just as you explored in chapter fourteen "The Law of Action." Victoria took three steps toward change: See it. **Feel** it. Do it.

By aligning herself with people like Tanya and Greg, Victoria had people to **Follow** as her models. Their like-mindedness provided her with support and their positivity encouraged her to keep moving **Forward**.

In the end, Victoria got even more than she thought possible—the childhood dream she had long since given up on became a reality.

CHAPTER
22

DREAM BIG!

Shoot for the stars—you are worth it! Or as a **Friend** of mine says: "Shoot for the moon and even if you don't quite make it, you could land on a star where you can rest and regroup for your next shot at the moon." Regardless of which you prefer, the message is the same—GO BIG!

> *If your dreams don't scare you, they may not be big enough!*

Remember when you were a child and the things you wanted to do in life ranged from really simple and close to home right through to those very lofty goals that would take your far from your safe haven of home and **Family**? The little things you dreamt of were in large part about being in the moment and, in their own way, they were big too. It was facing your fear as you achieved those little goals that helped you grow the confidence that would carry you into action toward your bigger dreams.

Perhaps you wanted to go down the giant slide at the park or to go higher than you'd ever gone before on the swing. Both of these are big dreams in the context of a small child. Or maybe you wanted to play outside with your **Friends** after dark and the idea of staying up late was thrilling. You were clearly stretching the boundaries and shooting for the stars in the context of a child's worldview.

It is possible that by the time you were ten your dreams had evolved a little to be more **Future Focused**. Some of them were huge but you weren't daunted by that. You simply knew that you were interested in **Following** that path to your dream. Some of us wanted to be movie stars and others were determined to uncover the next great find as an archaeologist. On a Monday, Johnny might have dreamt of being a doctor and by Friday, he was definitely going to be a fireman.

It's been said by researchers that the dreams we had when we were ten years old are likely still the same dreams we have today. If we're able to remember that far back and if we're honest enough with ourselves to admit that we might have known more at ten than we do today, it could be a topic worth exploring. Perhaps it's not the literal dream that still rings true for you. If you break that ten-year-old's dream down into elements, you might just find your adult dream buried there too.

Dreaming big doesn't mean that you have to wait till you achieve your ultimate goal before you celebrate. The journey is worthy of recognition too and there will be plenty of milestones and successes along the way to acknowledge. Dreaming big means that you've always got something to aim for. You'll always keep moving **Forward** and never **Feel** lost. Dreaming big doesn't mean that you have to have all the answers right at the outset and it doesn't mean that you can't ever change your mind. It just means that you've got somewhere important to go. It's more like a major journey, not a little trip around the block and to make that major journey you have to take several little trips around the block.

Simply put, it is just five little words so "Dream big and **Focus** small" and you'll get there every time!

What were some of your childhood dreams?

_____

_____

_____

_____

_____

Do they cross over into your adult goals? If so, how?

_____

_____

_____

_____

_____

How does it **Feel** to think about those childhood dreams again?

_____

_____

_____

_____

Which of your values and beliefs are supported by those childhood dreams?

_____

_____

_____

_____

What, if anything, might you do to reconnect with those childhood dreams?

_____

_____

_____

_____

What skills did you draw on to get creative in linking your childhood dreams with your goals as an adult?

_____

_____

_____

_____

How might you use those same skills to reframe other challenging questions you're **Facing** in your life right now?

_____

_____

_____

_____

How did those values and beliefs you identified a minute ago factor into your ability to reframe either the dream to the goal or the challenging question you are **Facing**?

_____

_____

_____

_____

What, if anything, will you do differently now that you've recalled these values and beliefs you carry?

_____

_____

_____

_____

_____

When will you do it?

_____

_____

_____

_____

"If opportunity doesn't knock, build a door."
Milton Berle

CHAPTER
23

EMBRACE THE FEAR

Fear is wound around and between most things we **Face** in life—including self-care. It can stop us in our tracks or it can propel us **Forward**. It is possible that our fear is logical and primal (by protecting us from life-threatening danger). More often, though, it makes little sense and doesn't really serve us. This is when we can draw on our **Friends** for support and perspective. "**Friends**" is one of those Really Great **F** Words—"fear" in its worst form is NOT, unless we can harness that fear and get it to work in our favour. If we can do that, then "fear" too can become a Really Great **F** Word. In **Fact**, I think I will make that happen right now—Abracadabra!—"**Fear**" is now one of the "good guys."

Many things start with **Fear** and most times **Fear** is what stops us from moving **Forward** to achieve our goals and dreams. Think of a time when **Fear** got in the way of your moving **Forward**. Perhaps it was a time when you were quite young and too shy to participate in an activity or a party you really wanted to attend. Maybe it was the **Fear** of failure that blocked you from trying for that promotion at work or the **Fear** of being turned down that got in the way of your asking that special someone out on a date.

All of us have endless examples that tell the story of being blocked by **Fear**. Susan Jeffers, Ph.D., encourages us to "**Feel** the **Fear** and Do It Anyway" in her book of the same name (1986). Jeffers breaks **Fear** down into something that has motivated readers for decades, and their shift to "Doing It Anyway" can be the torch that lights the way for the rest of us to **Follow**.

When I think of those occasions when I've punched through my **Fear** and moved to action, I realize that there were times when my move to action may have been the result of my **Fear** of staying where I was being greater than my **Fear** of moving **Forward**! How ironic is that? Thankfully, whatever the motivation, I did move to action and I also lived to tell the tale, which in the end gives me both the confidence and experience to draw on, the next time I'm faced with a similar **Fear** or barrier.

Making our **Fear** work for us is a goal and I know that when I want to achieve a goal I need to be intentional about moving to action. Even though, as I've said, **Fear** can occasionally leave me **Feeling** paralyzed and stuck, I know I need to move **Forward** and so I do. Many times my **Fear** is nothing more than my negative self-talk trying to block me from moving toward my goal(s). These are the times when I am thankful for the strategies I have intentionally put into place. It is those strategies that I draw on to manage my negative self-talk and to support me to move to action in spite of my **Fear**. (See your own list of strategies in chapter four "Beating the Bad.")

As was the case for Victoria in the preceding story, hope is a legitimate and powerful strategy. Quite possibly, it is the antidote for the worst kind of **Fear**, and something that will help provide a **Foundation** for the courage needed to lean **Forward** into **Fear**.

In a recent conversation, one of my clients said, "I think I'm the same as most people: I need to have hope as the carrot that keeps me motivated to take one more step **Forward**."

That client is a hundred percent correct—she is the same as most of us. The belief that our goal is achievable and the hope that we can make it there are instrumental to our success.

Another way we can move in the direction of making our **Fear** work for us is to "Fake it till you are it." The intention behind these words is different from the expression you may have previously heard, "Fake it till you make it." "Fake it till you are it" is the powerful message that Harvard professor and social psychologist Amy Cuddy delivers at a global TED Talk in 2012.[2] Her message of how

---

[2] ted.com/talks/amy_cuddy_your_body_language_shapes_who_you_are

our body language affects not only how we are perceived by others but also how we see ourselves is thought provoking. Cuddy describes the science behind physiological changes in our bodies and brains as we intentionally adjust our body language. The relevance of this interesting reality to our own practice of self-care is powerful. If adjusting the position of the way we sit or stand can change the chemical make-up of our brains then why wouldn't practising self-care, even when we're forcing ourselves to do it, help create a new reality in which self-care becomes second nature? I encourage you to view Amy's TED Talk and decide for yourself.

TED Talks are something you may want to consider incorporating into your regular self-care practice. They're available online and I always Feel good after listening to one that appeals to me. For me, time with TED Talks is time well spent. They're also a great excuse to get together with Friends. As a group, you can view a TED Talk and then spend the next hour or two in Focused Conversation about the topic. This is a stimulating, educational, and Fun way to give yourself an extra dose of self-care.

Fear is real for all of us. My choice is to make **Fear** work for me in support of my goals. I know that when I'm able to get the butterflies in my stomach—the ones that often accompany nervous anxiety—to fly in **Formation** versus flitting about helter skelter, I am well on my way to achieving my goal. Having **Focused** conversations with **Friends** is one way that I put my **Fear** into perspective. **Following** the rule of chapter sixteen "Begin *Before* You're Ready" also helps me beat **Fear**. That new perspective and my intentional move to action help me see the hope clearly, which encourages me to embrace my **Fear** as I do the dance of life. It is also the way that I turn **Fear** into a Really Good **F** Word on a regular basis.

    This interactive book, your community of **Friends**, and the **Focused** conversations you've engaged in have all supported you in developing strategies and an action plan for self-care. That same process can be used for any topic. As you've engaged in some of the activities and conversations, you may have **Felt** some level of discomfort (*aka* **Fear**). Somehow you were able to **Feel** the **Fear** and do it anyway—congratulations!

What other times in your life have you overcome **Fear** and moved to action?

_____

_____

_____

_____

_____

What did you do or use to be able to overcome that **Fear**?

_____

_____

_____

_____

How will you use this knowledge to help you the next time you **Feel** held back by **Fear?**

_____

_____

_____

_____

_____

What might get in the way of your success?

_____

_____

_____

_____

What will you do to overcome those hurdles?

_____

_____

_____

_____

"Wisdom is like a new kind of womb."
Marianne Williamson

Group Activity #8

Here is a two-part activity for your next **Fun-Filled** get-together. Use your small-group time in Part One to brainstorm with your **Friends**. By starting this conversation in the small group, everyone will have the opportunity to be **Fully** engaged. By doing this with your **Friends**, as opposed to on your own, you will be able to ask one another questions that will help with recalling situations that reflect the questions. You'll also be able to come up with specific examples you can use once you get into the large-group discussion in Part Two.

Part One: In groups of two or three people, discuss examples where **Fear** has been a **Factor** in stopping you or encouraging you to move **Forward**. Come up with your own questions for the discussion. Some of mine might be, "Did hope play a role in those examples at all? If so, what role did it play? If you could have a do-over, what might you do differently next time? Where would you find the courage and skill to face the **Fear** and make it work for you? Have you ever had a 'Fake it till you are it' experience? How did it change you in the long term?"

Remember, you can make up your own questions to support your partner(s). Lend your **Friends** your curiosity and your ability to actively listen to help them hear themselves.

Part Two: Return to the larger group and continue the discussion sharing your insights and examples from the small groups. Take the time to ensure everyone participates in this large group experience.

CHAPTER
24

REWRITE THE RULES!

If we have the power to turn **Fear** into a really good **F** word that works for us rather than against us, what other rules might we be able to rewrite? Could we create a reality in which stress and anxiety **Feed** us as opposed to leaving us **Feeling** drained and exhausted?

Perhaps just saying "yes" might be an answer or at least a step toward rewriting rules. When I **Feel** hesitant about moving **Forward** because of an old belief or rule, I wonder if it's as important to understand where the rule originated or if all I need to do is recognize that it exists and then combat it with a simple "yes" instead of the "no" that is screaming to get out. This ties back into chapter four "Beating the Bad," where we **Focused** on stories, examples, and strategies for defeating negative self-talk. It is also linked to the cookie-jar concept. We know that if we're practising healthy (and regular) self-care—enough that our jar is **Full** all the time—we will be in a position to **Feel** empowered and confident about rewriting any rules that are not serving us. Negative self-talk and rules that don't serve us are very often linked together.

"When we listen to our intuition, embrace all of our imperfections, and stay authentic to who we are, this is taking care."
Cat Li Stevenson

Some of the rules we've accumulated throughout our lives serve us very well and others don't. In the same way that you clean out your closet to make room for new clothes at the start of a different season, we need to get rid of old rules (or rewrite them) to ensure they're serving us in moving toward whatever it is we want. Basically, if your rules are no longer serving you and your dreams—it's time to make room for new ones.

Those rules act like **Filters**—**Filters** that we view everything through and that affect the way we behave, the choices we make, and the beliefs we go **Forward** with. You change the **Filter** in your furnace regularly. How often do you check or change the **Filters** in your mind?

What are some of those rules or **Filters** you'd like to rewrite (or let go of)?

_____

_____

_____

_____

_____

How do those rules or **Filters** affect your beliefs/behaviour/choices?

_____

_____

_____

_____

How will you rewrite them?

_____

_____

_____

_____

What might get in the way of **Following** the new rules or using the new **Filters**?

_____

_____

_____

_____

How will you support yourself to adhere to the new way of thinking?

_____

_____

_____

_____

What are some of the old rules and filters that drive our choices today? I've come up with a few and included some of my thoughts on them. How many more can you come up with? What thoughts will you add to the ones I've listed? Perhaps this will be another conversation for one of your gatherings of great **Friends**?

Old Rule #1: "Children should be seen and not heard."

Really? It seems to me that the qualities that drive us crazy in kids are the ones we most admire in adults.

Old Rule #2: "Don't brag."

When does celebrating cross the line to become bragging? Is this simply another skill that we need practise to master? If we want to be good at a sport, an activity, or at interpersonal skills like conflict resolution or coaching, we know we need to practise. How are talents like knowing when celebration turns into unhealthy bragging any different?

Old Rule #3: "Be careful."

> *Said too many times, this rule might create an adult who is afraid to take the necessary risks required to live a rich <u>Full</u> life.*

Old Rule #4: "You made your bed; now you must lie in it."

> *True to some degree. I do however get to remake my bed every time I get up!*

Old Rule #5: "It's women's (men's) work."

> *Not in my world.*

186

Old Rule #6: "Life is not a bed of roses."

> *That's okay, because I prefer carnations.*

What are some other old "rules" or "**Filters**" you've heard? What are your thoughts about them and how might they be re-framed to be a better fit for the world we live in today?

_____

_____

_____

_____

_____

_____

Rules and **Filters** such as these are typically imposed by the culture we live in (cultural norms). They may have been impressed upon us in our youth by **Family**, **Friends**, and school or life experiences. In **Fact**, a common term for many of the rules and **Filters** we live by is "parent tapes." That's not to say that they just came from our parents; they simply came to us during a formative time in our lives. There is no doubt that they were well-intentioned and of value at one time. When we begin to take a closer look and evaluate the **Filters** we use in making our adult decisions, there can sometimes be opportunity for growth through **Forging** new paths and rewriting the rules.

"I'm not wasting time. I'm not being lazy. I'm taking care of me."
Kimberly Mackereth

CHAPTER
25

DISCONNECT TO
RECONNECT

When was the last time that you were able to truly disconnect from technology? Unplug the computer, cancel the cable, and turn off the phone. What if there were no Facebook, no need to keep up with the tweets, and your inbox was empty? How many more hours would you have available to reconnect with the **Friends** and **Family** who are right there in your home or just down the street? How much more time would you choose to spend on your own self-care? What would you do with that time? Please be as honest and specific as possible as you think about these questions. Your next Personal Assignment and Group Activity will **Focus** on them.

While it may not be realistic to think we can take this aggressive a stance in eliminating technology while still maintaining our careers and long-distance relationships, I challenge you to actually consider how far you could go on this path before you'd be putting your life as you need it to be at risk. Could you unplug for an hour a day? What about committing to turn everything off at a specific time each evening? What would happen if even a half day on the weekend was **Free** of technology?

A few years ago, I was working with a very large organization that was extremely bureaucratic in its structure. As is typical of every bureaucracy I've ever been affiliated with, technology played a huge role in its daily business practices. Email was the preferred method of communicating and everyone's inbox was filled to overflowing every time they checked it. Virtual meetings were commonplace and intended to save both time and money. Everyone from middle management upward in the hierarchy was assigned a cell phone and expected to be available for emergencies 24/7. It is safe to say that they were so reliant on technology that if the power went out, staff would experience a significant sense of inability to do their work.

My role with this organization was to develop training initiatives for leadership skills, interpersonal communication, conflict resolution, and stress management. As I did my research for expected learning outcomes, current practices in each of these areas, and levels of employee engagement, I came across one department in the organization where employees seemed to be more engaged, less stressed, and happier overall.

The only difference I was able to uncover was that this one little department had made a decision to intentionally disconnect their technology (as best they could) every Friday. As a department, they had committed to practising some self-care by making Fridays email-free days. Instead, they chose to pick up the phone or walk down the hall and connect with their colleagues in a way that would put the human element back into their interactions.

I wish I could say that the rest of this large organization chose to **Follow** their lead and learn from the experience of that one little department. Unfortunately, as is often the case in big business, that was not the outcome. I'm a sucker for the little guy and I love it when someone or a group is able to rise above the status quo to find a better place. My sincere hope is that this little department is still being intentional about its self-care and that its members will continue to behave like David in the face of Goliath.

Personal Assignment #4

If you haven't already done it, set aside at least thirty minutes to consider how you would respond to the questions that I've scattered throughout chapter twenty-five. Write down your answers. What other questions do you think it is important to ask on this topic?

What would you disconnect **First** and why?

_____

_____

_____

_____

Research technology-based addictions and consider your own behaviours with social media and other technology.

_____

_____

_____

_____

What are your thoughts about the little department that acted like David in the face of its Goliath?

_____

_____

_____

_____

Where in your life have you or could you behave like this example of David?

_____

_____

_____

_____

How do these questions about breaking from the status quo leave you **Feeling**?

_____

_____

_____

_____

_____

Group Activity #9

Discuss your findings and personal insights with the rest of your group. Are there common themes? How much of a role do personal values play in an individual's decision about how far they would go in unplugging from communication technology? What about the demographics of your group? Do age, socioeconomic status, or life experience **Factor** into people's decisions?

CHAPTER 26

THERE IS NOTHING NEW IN THE WORLD

"If we keep doing what we've always done, we'll continue to get what we've always got." Or another way to say the same thing is, "Nothing will change unless something changes." We've all heard these words of wisdom or at least something that sounds very much like them. It seems as though it should be an easy concept to grasp and incorporate into our lives. Yet for some reason it is a lesson that can be difficult to learn. In **Fact**, it is a lesson that many of us need to revisit regularly.

Typically, these words of wisdom are uttered in conjunction with a behaviour that is not serving us in moving **Forward** to the place where we want to be. In keeping with the spirit of appreciative inquiry though, these same words can also be flipped on their heads and reframed to bring **Focus** to behaviours that are working for us. ("Appreciative inquiry" is a popular leadership strategy that you might want to Google. Since you are the CEO of yourself, it might be a concept you'd like to explore further in support of your own growth.)

I'm often amazed by the **Fact** that so many of us are willing to abandon behaviours that have been bringing us success. And to make it an even more intriguing concept, we often let go of them at the same time as we seem to be making the greatest advances on a goal we've been working toward. We are interesting creatures!

Can you think of a time when you've sabotaged your own success? I can think of a couple of examples for myself. Most common are my exercise goals. I always begin with the best of intentions and do a great job of staying on track with my plan until the novelty wears off and I begin to see success. Interestingly, it is right at the point when I know I'm making progress and I start to **Feel** stronger that I fall back into old habits. Those old habits include "doing it later," and for those of you who can empathize with this you'll know that my "later" turns into "much later" and eventually "never," until I climb back on the wagon and begin again.

It is my commitment to self-care that has taught me to pay attention to my cookie jar. It is my self-awareness and those wise words about "Nothing changes unless something changes" that prompt me to climb back on the wagon where my exercise goals are intentional and a priority. And it is my self-care practice that enables me to **Forgive** myself, knowing that every day is a new day, and to begin again.

Personal Assignment #5

Bring a pen and paper to a quiet place and plan to take at least thirty minutes to **Fast Forward** your life. Consider the wisdom in "If I keep doing what I've always done, I'll get what I've always got." Overlay that wisdom on your life. Journal about how these wise words are reflected in your life and what you might do to use the concept in support of your goal for increased self-care.

If you ever find yourself stuck in your journaling process, try switching hands. Sometimes writing with your non-dominant hand can prompt new perspective and get the ink flowing again.

Group Activity #10

Part One: In small groups of two or three, discuss how this journaling exercise supports your own self-awareness. Plan to give each person in your small group a minimum of fifteen minutes of **Focused** time and attention. As you listen to your partner(s), be intentional with the questions you ask one another. Frame your questions so they begin with the words "what" and "how" as best you can, as that will support your **Friends** in deepening their own self-awareness.

Part Two: Return to the large group and facilitate a discussion where everyone has an opportunity to share their experience and their learning.

"Enjoy life; there are no reruns."
Unknown

CHAPTER
27

SUFFERING IS OPTIONAL

What's the thing that will call you to action? This is a key question for the activities in this chapter. We've all heard ourselves and others refer to things we "have to do." I encourage you to challenge yourself on that statement. Anything that we do, even when it isn't serving us, is our choice. If it's a choice that is causing us to suffer, perhaps it's time to take a closer look.

Some of us will choose to wait until a serious illness strikes, or an important relationship breaks down. Others of us will choose to pay attention to the early warning signs. Which will you choose?

There is a parable that I often share with clients whom I suspect may not be paying attention to the early warning signs and instead are choosing to suffer through self-assigned obligations. This parable is a great demonstration of the deceptive nature of stress and how important it is to pay attention to those early warning signs. I share the parable and then ask the client "How does that speak to you?" They always have an answer as we all know our own truth.

A frog is dropped into a pot of boiling water and he jumps right back out. He is then put into a pot of cool water, which is set upon the stove at a low heat. The frog swims around in his pot of tepid water very happily. Eventually the water heats and tepid turns to boiling but the frog never jumps out ... he just swims around in there till it's too late. Unknowingly that frog adjusted to the gradual warming of the water and before he knew what happened he had waited too long and was cooked.

The moral of this story is found in the insidious nature of the gradually warming water in the pot. It is exactly the same as what happens to all of us in our daily lives if we aren't self-aware and practising healthy self-care regularly and on purpose. Often we don't admit how tired we are until it's too late and we end up sick in bed. Other times we don't want to acknowledge how stressed or unhappy we are in a specific situation until it's too late. Hopefully, the result is nothing too serious.

Unfortunately, the reality is that all too often this extreme level of stress manifests in a heart attack or another serious illness.

By paying attention to how hot the water is on a regular basis, we will be well positioned to recognize when it begins to warm rather than waiting till it's too late to get out. The way to continually check the temperature of the water in your pot is to use the analogy of the cookie jar. Be intentional about evaluating the state of your cookie jar and taking the time to bake cookies on a regular basis.

Personal Assignment #6

Set aside an hour of uninterrupted time for yourself. Google "self-care inventories" and other self-care research materials online. Once you've located an inventory or some reading material that appeals to you, read it, do it, evaluate your response to it, and spend a minimum of ten minutes journaling about how your self-awareness has been enhanced. Do your best to include some written commitment to adjust any choices you're currently making that are not serving your life.

Group Activity #11

Part One: In small groups of two or three, brainstorm two lists. One list will include the early warning signs of the consequences to "suffering" and the other list will include more serious scenarios—when early warning signs have been ignored. Everything on these lists will be examples of a life event or behaviour that might call you to action in choosing to initiate a change.

Part Two: Return to the large group and share your lists with your **Friends**. Discuss how this activity ties into Group Activity #10. Provide an opportunity for everyone in the large group to share their biggest take-away from this activity.

CHAPTER
28

EVERYBODY DESERVES A COACH!

At the very beginning of this book I explained that coaches help create a perfect storm for their clients. A coach's perfect storm is where passion and desire meet planning, preparation, and commitment to action. My intention in writing this book is to provide you with stories, information, activities, and intentional questions that open the door to answers that best inform your next steps as you strategize for success in achieving your self-care goal(s).

As you reflect back over the process, I hope you will say that you found yourself thinking in new ways, that you've **Felt** challenged on occasion, and that you've **Felt** heard and understood along the way. I hope too that you will have experienced how the coaching process can be a powerful tool in the practice of intentional self-care.

Another thing that we did over the course of this book is we created your community of support in chapter twelve: "My **Favourite F** Words." In your Group Activities, you constructed a confidential environment built on norms such as mutual respect and willingness to participate through both sharing and listening. That community of support has been **Filling** the role of coach throughout this book. You may have discovered that this community of support is a perfect match for you in continuing your intentional practice of self-care and you will continue to meet long after you've read the final pages of this book. Remember, though, you will always have the book to refer back to and refresh, revitalize, or rebuild your community of support at any time.

Self-care is not the only topic that coaching is used for. As an executive coach, I find my clients' interests range from strategizing for purely business goals to coaching for personal objectives and life dreams. For those of you who are interested in working with a coach, here are my suggestions as you move along that path.

Finding the coach who is the best match for you is important, so if you decide you'd like to explore what it would be like to work with a coach on a regular basis I encourage you to **Follow** these six simple steps.

1. Choose two or three coaches to interview. Check out their websites and references as you create this shortlist of possible candidates. Remember, you're hiring an important member of your personal team, so go into this process like an employer.

2. Expect prospective coaches to be willing to give you a complimentary sample session (usually about ten to fifteen minutes).

3. Look for someone you **Feel** you can connect with. This intangible vibe is difficult to describe; we all know when we're attracted to someone and we also know when we are not. You will need to **Feel** as though you can trust your coach a hundred percent of the time. Remember, they will be your confidential nonjudgmental thinking partner so you need to **Feel** completely secure in their ability to keep your confidence.

4. Expect to commit to a minimum term contract with your coach. (Most often, I ask clients to commit to at least three months of meetings twice monthly, i.e. six sessions over a long enough period of time to achieve results.) Most coaches will require a minimum commitment from their clients. That commitment speaks to a client's readiness to engage in the coaching process and her willingness to move to action on her goals.

5. Ask prospective coaches questions about what they expect from their clients. This question will give you good insight into a potential coach's philosophy.

6. Ultimately, trust your intuition.

> *Most coaches will work either face to face or at a distance using a variety of technology, so don't <u>Feel</u> your options are limited if you live in a remote location. I have clients from all over North America who connect with me via Skype, FaceTime, telephone, and in person.*

Personal Assignment #7

Identify a personal goal, aspiration, or commitment that you'd like to work toward. The sky is the limit. Get really clear on what your goal is. You can use any topic—work related or personal. Write it down.

_____

_____

_____

_____

Consider what is standing in the way of your achieving that goal. Write down those barriers.

_____

_____

_____

_____

Which of those barriers are you currently tolerating?

_____

_____

_____

_____

How does it **Feel** when you hear yourself identify the barriers that you're tolerating?

_____

_____

_____

_____

_____

What would it take for you to decide that you're no longer prepared to tolerate them?

_____

_____

_____

_____

How committed are you to making changes?

_____

_____

_____

_____

What do you need to do as a **First** step toward making those changes?

_____

_____

_____

_____

What might get in the way of your **First** step?

_____

_____

_____

_____

_____

Think of a time when you've overcome a similar barrier in the past. What did you do that time? What did you draw on to be able to overcome it?

_____

_____

_____

_____

_____

How might that experience help you in this scenario?

_____

_____

_____

_____

How prepared do you **Feel** to move **Forward** in taking that **First** step right now?

_____

_____

_____

_____

When will you take it?

_____

_____

_____

_____

How will you hold yourself accountable to taking that **First** step?

_____

_____

_____

_____

These last few questions demonstrate what it would be like to work with your coach on a topic of your choosing. It is their job to keep you moving **Forward** in the direction of your goal. They will draw out your answers and use your past successes to support you in reaching your target. Your coach will believe that you absolutely CAN do anything you want to do and they will do their best in support of you getting where you want to go.

Personal Assignment #8

Ask ten people to describe some of your greatest strengths. Write them all down. Look for common themes. Be a detective and uncover evidence that demonstrates the skills you've used in the past and the successes you've had that have led to those strengths being identified by people who know you. It's important to stick to the **Facts** as you go through this process. The **Facts** will fortify the evidence. Don't rush through this activity—you've earned the good **Feeling** that comes with recognizing who you are.

Group Activity #12

This group activity is based on the work you did in personal assignment #8. Depending on the number of people in your group, you might need to spread this activity over more than one get-to-gether. If your gatherings are anything like mine, the social aspect and the very important **Fun** take up a good portion of the time. When I did this activity with my **Friends**, we chose to have two or three people share their findings at each gathering. That meant that we had an excellent excuse to get together at least four times just for this one activity!

Plan to give each person in your group ten to fifteen minutes to share their top ten strengths and the evidence they've come up with to support those observations from the people of whom they asked the question.

At the end of each person's turn, have the rest of the large group brainstorm additional evidence for those top ten strengths and have the person include them on their written list of factual evidence.

Personal Assignment #9

This assignment is like having a garden. It is both **Future Focused** in that you will be planting seeds and at the same time, you will be paying attention to appreciating the bounty that is already right in **Front** of you.

Part One: Come up with ideas and opportunities for yourself to grow. Perhaps you'll have a health-related goal you'd like to **Focus** on. Maybe there is a new career move on the horizon or some education you've been considering. What about that person you've been avoiding—is there an opportunity to rewrite that story? Got a trip you'd like to plan and save for? Maybe some new appliances for the kitchen or new tires for the car? **Feel Free** to ask your **Friends** for help and advice with this list. This is the **Future Focused** planting of seeds in your garden. As you write down these ideas and opportunities, your subconscious will begin to visualize them. Down the road when you're ready to move to action on them, you'll already have that **Foundation** in place. Refer back to chapter fourteen "The Law of Action" where we talked about visualization as being the **First** step toward moving to action on achieving a goal.

Part Two: Take the time to identify and recognize your accomplishments to this day. Perhaps there is an example of a moment where you chose self-care over self-sacrifice, or maybe you made a decision that you still **Feel** good about. You might have made progress on a project, or even completed a task. Remember to make it about today. Stay as close to being in the moment with recognizing and celebrating your success as you can.

Part Three: Specifically, what did you do today to shift your thinking and reframe your negative thoughts into positive language? By paying attention to this, you will become even more intentional with the practice until eventually it becomes second nature for you.

Group Activity #13

In small groups of two or three, discuss the challenges and the outcome of Personal Assignment #9. Which parts of it were easiest for you? What was the most challenging? How do your answers to those questions inform you as you go **Forward**?

Use this small group setting to dig deeper into all three parts of this assignment. By this time, you will have come to know one another pretty well and your trust will be high enough for you to be completely honest as you help your **Friends** with their responses. As always, use "what" and "how" questions as you communicate in this respectful and thoughtful environment.

Group Activity #14

In your large group come up with ideas for **Future** gatherings. Keep the **Fun** alive. Keep your **Friends** close by. Maintain your **Focus**. Continue to lean **Forward** into your best life. And of course—don't forget the **Food**!

CHAPTER 29

IN THE BEGINNING, THERE WAS SELF-CARE AND IT WAS NOT SELFISH!

Congratulations! Perhaps this is an opportunity to reframe another **F** word into something that is really good. There are times when the word **Finished** can be interpreted as not so positive and there are other times that it **Feels** like a really good **F** word. How are you **Feeling** about the word "**Finished**" right now? You've made it to the end of this book and if you've done the work along the way, you're well on your way to achieving your goal of increased self-care. It may be the end of the book; however, it's just the beginning of your independent self-care journey and an opportunity for you to continue with the intentional work you've been engaged in. While it may seem overwhelming at times, remember to use those special ingredients in baking your cookies and **Filling** your cookie jar. Draw on the support of your **Friends** and **Family**, stay **Focused**, move **Forward**, and have **Fun**.

It can be a challenge to stay on track and recall these simple steps. That's because they may be simple and at the same time, not always easy; so be kind to yourself as you continue along this path.

Remember too that you're not alone. Many others are on a similar track and there is a lot of help available; you only need to be open to accepting it. This is where your support network, your coach, your action plan, and this book will aid you in achieving success.

Taking just one step at a time or breaking the big picture into small bite-sized pieces are important, so stick to your plan. You've taken the time to plan the plan, so now all you have to do is continue to **Follow** that plan, and ultimately the results really will take care of themselves. When we look at anything in its entirety, it often appears simply too large to manage. Broken down it becomes so much more doable.

Now that we really are at the end, the final few lines, it's incumbent on me as your coach, to push you a little, to encourage you to move to action, or maintain the momentum you've built during the work you've done with this book, and to help you hold yourself accountable. Call your network of **Friends** and set a date for your next gathering. If you skimmed through this book and thought that you'd do some of it later when you had more time, I remind you that the time is *now*, so go back to page one!

You picked up this book for a reason. Reflect on what that reason was and use it to move to action. Give yourself the gift you deserve and take the time today to continue your journey to increased self-care. With a little luck and some intentional choices, you may never hear yourself say, "If only I'd known then what I know now."

"I want to die young at a ripe old age."
Montague Francis Ashley-Montagu

Author Biography

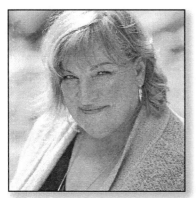

Lorrie Forde is a daughter, a mother, a sister, a grandma, and a friend. She learned the hard way that balance is her secret ingredient in the analogy of a full and healthy 'cookie jar'. During a twenty-five year career in post-secondary education and through her work as a professional Executive and Life Coach, Lorrie has gathered the research and the tools she needed to bring this book to life. "I believe everyone deserves to have a coach and this book was a way for me to make that possible. I invite my readers to have fun with the process and to trust that their answers will come—they always do." Lorrie loves to fill her days with adventure and laughter. She enjoys her work and says, "I work hard but I work to live—I don't live to work."

Author Information

Talk to me…

I'd love to hear about your experience with Really Good F Words. Send me your self-care stories and tell me about how you beat the negative self-talk that threatened to get in the way of you achieving your goal(s). What was your biggest take-away from the experience of working through this book and how will you maintain the momentum you've built over these pages? I look forward to hearing from you—please email me at lorrie@mountaintopcoaching.ca or follow me on Facebook, Twitter, Instagram, or Pinterest.

Being able to connect with my readers is important to me and receiving lots of reviews for my book is important to the book's success so please take a minute to visit my Author Page on Amazon. The link is www.amazon.com/author/lorrieforde From there you'll find a spot where you can Follow Me, where you can give Really Good F Words your review, and where you can see what events I have coming up. Who knows…maybe I'll be in a city near you and we'll have the opportunity to meet in person.

Lorrie Forde, CEC ACC
12819 Schaeffer Crescent
Summerland, BC V0H 1Z4
Canada
lorrie@mountaintopcoaching.ca
www.mountaintopcoaching.ca
www.facebook.com/mountaintopcoaching
twitter: @lorrief

Lorrie Forde is the founding owner of Mountaintop Coaching. She earned her designation of Certified Executive Coach at Royal Roads University in Victoria, British Columbia. This graduate certificate program is recognized world-wide. In addition to her coaching credential, Lorrie is also certified to administer the EQi and EQ360 tools that measure levels of emotional intelligence. Our emotional intelligence is the filter through which we see and are seen by the world around us. EQ (emotional intelligence) can be developed throughout life so it is a perfect partner for anyone coaching toward a goal.

Lorrie is an active member of the International Coach Federation (coachfederation.org) as well as her local chapter of the International Coach Federation in the Okanagan Valley of British Columbia, Canada. (icf-okanagan.org)

The work that Lorrie's clients bring to her coaching table is varied. Some of her clients are purely business focused and others of them are more interested in personal goals. Executives often retain her as their coach as they develop strategic plans for the coming year(s). Middle managers and supervisors at times access Lorrie to role play difficult conversations as they find the words that are "right" for them. Personal goals range from developing an intentional self-care practice through to transitioning from work to retirement. Bottom line is that, in coaching, the client is the boss and they get to choose whatever they'd like to focus on. Even when the client doesn't feel like the boss—Lorrie will help them find the words they're looking for. As their coach, she is there to support them and to use some really great questions that are designed to shine a light on new perspective. Throughout the coaching process Lorrie holds space for her client so they have room and time to uncover their own best answers. Lorrie describes herself as a confidential, non-judgemental thinking partner who shares her client's goal.

Lorrie also hosts retreats for her clients. These retreats include creating space for a bit of self-care at the same time as there is a schedule committed to customized private coaching on a topic of the client's choosing. If you'd like to work with Lorrie as your coach or experience one of her retreats all you have to do is contact her at the email above.

"No one needs a coach, but everybody deserves one!"
Lorrie Forde